365 YOGA

365 YOGA

Daily Meditations

JULIE RAPPAPORT

Jeremy P. Tarcher/Penguin
a member of Penguin Group (USA) Inc.
New York

Most Tarcher/Penguin books are available at special quantity discounts for bulk purchase for sales promotions, premiums, fund-raising, and educational needs. Special books or book excerpts also can be created to fit specific needs. For details, write Penguin Group (USA) Inc. Special Markets, 375 Hudson Street, New York, NY 10014.

Jeremy P. Tarcher/Penguin
a member of
Penguin Group (USA) Inc.
375 Hudson Street
New York, NY 10014
www.penguin.com

Library of Congress Cataloging-in-Publication Data

Rappaport, Julie, date.
365 yoga : daily meditations / Julie Rappaport.
p. cm.
Includes bibliographical references.
ISBN 1-58542-324-6
1. Yoga. 2. Spiritual life—Meditations. I. Title.
BL1238.52.R4 2004 2003071157
204'.36—dc22

Printed in the United States of America
1 3 5 7 9 10 8 6 4 2

BOOK DESIGN BY JENNIFER ANN DADDIO

I dedicate this book

TO PEACE FOR ALL BEINGS EVERYWHERE.

Om Shanti, Shanti, Shanti!

Om Peace, Peace, Peace!

LIFE'S LONGING
FOR ITSELF

Yoga is happening right now. It is Now. And it is simpler than you think. Through yoga we dive straight into the heart of life and into what lives inside of us. We feel this in our pores; in our muscles, bones, and breath. We feel our connection to all that "Is" and we have direct experience of this "Isness" every time we connect our body to our breath. Borrowing a phrase from the poet Kahlil Gibran, yoga is simply a most fundamental and intimate expression of *life's longing for itself*; we are the life, the love, and the joy that we seek.

Nothing external is required to enter into yoga. Not even the daily teachings in this book. The words that you find here are simply meant to act as a living teacher would: to help you find clarity and to serve as a guide or mirror, on your journey with yoga and with all of life. More important than any text or any teaching is your relationship with your own body, breath, and mind—with your own true Self. When authentic body-mind integration occurs, a wholeness emerges that leads us toward profound peace. This is yoga.

Striking a balance between action and reflection could be considered one of the goals of yoga. Is it more important to engage with the practices of yoga or with the philosophy? To practice without awareness will block any real transformation, yet the danger with too much philosophy is the tendency toward abstraction and intellectualization. As the great sage Vasistha says: "If you conceptualize this teaching for your intellectual entertainment and do not let it act in your own life, you will stumble and fall like a blind man." I offer the passages in this volume as tools for both PRACTICE and reflection. With these tools we may take yoga to deeper levels of understanding. Then our living practice will become luminous and clear the path toward enlightenment.

Writing about yoga presents a few obstacles. Naming the Nameless is a bit like trying to catch soap bubbles in your hand: enticing but impossible. In assembling *365 Yoga* I have had the privilege to delve directly into sacred spiritual texts from many traditions and to surround myself with yogic and universal wisdom that touches me. I have been moved to write my own meditations on yoga, which are sprinkled throughout the book. This living tradition grows each day, and I hope the ancient and modern texts that I have chosen reflect this evolution and encourage both those new to yoga and seasoned practitioners to look deeply into themselves and their yoga. I hope that these collected texts accurately transmit the vitality and diversity of yoga, which is like the cosmic serpent Ananta: limitless and infinitely transformative.

Some ways to utilize this book: Read one selection per day, before or after your home practice or yoga class, try out some of the practices that I offer, or flip through the book and read what grabs you. Let these meditations act as an organizing principle. Read a quote in the morning before work or in the evening before sleep. Try closing your eyes and opening a page at random. Or write your own reflections on yoga.

You, the reader, are not asked to buy into any one of the views presented here but to sample from the multiplicity of perspectives. For those who feel a bit overwhelmed by the philosophical underpinnings of this vast tradition, I hope that the selected texts from both East and West will introduce you to the beautiful poetry and prose that spring from the depths of mystical experience. If most of your experience with yoga has been through the practice of physical postures (asanas) in isolation from the sacred teachings, my sincere wish is to show how yoga can work as a spiritual and relevant force in your life.

I hope these pages will inspire you to practice and that some of these teachings will touch you and lead you into the grace of yoga, which is the grace of the divine energy living in all of us, as us.

OM Shanti, Shanti, Shanti.
OM Peace, Peace, Peace.

I.

INVOCATION TO PATANJALI

Yogena cittasya padena vacam
Malamsarirasya ca vaidyakena
Yopakarottam pravaram muninam
Patanjalim pranjalirana tosmi

Ababu purushakaram
Sankhacakrasidharinam
Sahasrasirasam svetam
Pranamami Patanjalim

Shrimate Anataya Nagarajaya
Namo Namah

To the noblest of sages, Patanjali.
Who gave Yoga for serenity of mind,
Grammar for purity of speech,
And Medicine for perfection of the body, I bow.
I prostrate before Patanjali
Whose upper body has a human form,
Whose arms hold a conch and and disc,

Who is crowned by a thousand-headed cobra,
O incarnation of Adisesa, my salutations to thee.

THE BHOJAVRTTI

2.

Who am I who speaks, walks, stands, and functions on this elaborate stage known as the world? I should find this out.

YOGA VASISHTA

3.

PEACE INVOCATION FOR STUDY

Om saha navavatu. Saha nau bhunaktu.
Saha viryam karavavahai. Tejasvinavadhitamastu
Ma vidvisavahai
Om Shanti, Shanti, Shanti!

TAITTIRIYA UPANISHAD

Om. May we both be protected. May we both enjoy the
fruits of scriptual study. May we both exert together to
find the true meaning of the sacred text. May our studies
be fruitful. May we never quarrel with each other.
Om Peace, Peace Peace!

JR

4.

The Yoga we practice is not for ourselves alone, but for the Divine; its aim is to work out the will of the Divine in the world, to effect a spiritual transformation and to bring down a divine nature and a divine into the mental, vital, and physical nature and life of humanity.

Its object is not personal Mukti, although Mukti is a necessary condition of the Yoga, but the liberation and transformation of the human being.

SRI AUROBINDO

5.

Wisdom tells me I am nothing.
Love tells me I am everything.
And between the two my life flows.

SRI NISARGADATTA MAHARAJ

Om Gum Ganapatayei Namaha
Om and Salutation to the remover of obstacles for which
Gum is the seed.

GANESHA MANTRA

Before beginning any new endeavor invoking the elephant-headed
God, Ganesha/Ganapatayei, will ensure success. He is the remover of all obstacles and a potent symbol for the practice of
yoga.

JR

Hatha yoga is a refuge for all those who are scorched by the three
fires. To those who practice yoga, hatha yoga is like the tortoise
who supports the three worlds.

HATHA YOGA PRADIPIKA

BE YOGA

Lately, everywhere I turn people seem interested in yoga. "Do you 'do' yoga?" they ask.

"How long have you been doing yoga? What kind of yoga do you do?"

When you start "doing" yoga, you miss it all together. It becomes another pastime, rather than a way of being. Try living yoga, being yoga, and notice the difference between doing and being.

JR

By soul I mean, first of all, a perspective rather than a substance, a viewpoint toward things rather than a thing itself. This perspective is reflective; it mediates events and makes differences between ourselves and everything that happens. Between us and events, between the doer and the deed, there is a reflective moment—and soul-making means differentiating this middle ground.

JAMES HILLMAN

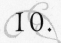

In your body is Mount Meru encircled by the seven continents; the rivers are there too, the seas, the mountains, the plains, and the gods of the fields. Prophets are to be seen in it, monks, places of pilgrimage and the deities presiding over them. The stars are there, and the planets, and the sun together with the moon; there too are the two cosmic forces: that which destroys, that which creates; and all the elements: ether, air and fire, water and earth. Yes, in your body are all things that exist in the three worlds, all performing their prescribed functions around Mount Meru. He alone who knows this is held to be a true yogi.

SIVA SAMHITA

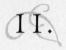

II.

Practicing yoga without clear attention to the breath is like trying to grow a plant without giving it water.

JR

12.

We have the feeling that every step of the path we tread should be a lotus and we develop a logic that interprets whatever happens to us accordingly. If we fall, we create a soft landing which prevents sudden shock. Surrendering does not involve preparing for a soft landing; it means just landing on hard, ordinary ground—on rocky, wild countryside. Once we open ourselves, then we land on what is.

CHOGYAM TRUNGPA

13.

Now is set forth the authoritive teaching on yoga.
Yoga is the ability to direct and focus mental activity.
With the attainment of focused mind, the inner being
establishes itself in all its reality.

YOGA SUTRA OF PATANJALI I:1–3

14.

BAKASANA—CRANE POSE

Cranes perch, birds fly.
Winding up for takeoff, transform your body into a high-
flying bird.
Thoughts cease in that second of pure consciousness, in that
moment of blissful flight.

Using your arms as pillars to hold up the temple of your
    body,
Come in for the landing and let your mind become the
Shelter of a million beautiful things.
Weightless weight pours into glistening claws—like hands
    balancing on solid earth, firm and free.

JR

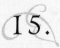

15.

However men try to reach me, I return their love with my love,
whatever path they may travel, it leads to me in the end.

BHAGAVAD GITA 4:11

16.

NATARAJASANA — SHIVA'S COSMIC DANCE

As the Hindu deity who most fully represents the ascetic's journey, the god Shiva is an apt mirror for aspiring yogis. A renunciate with wild hair, consort of the goddesses Parvati and Ganga, Shiva resides for thousands of years meditating in his Himalayan cave. One of the three major Hindu gods, Shiva contains both masculine and feminine attributes. While all the gods have a hand in manifesting the universe, Shiva also destroys that which binds us to material existence. When not meditating in his Himalayan cave, Shiva can be found dancing in the temples. Through his ecstatic dance of creation and destruction, he becomes the holder of the universe while balancing on one leg. In natarajasana (the pose of Shiva) the uplifted leg represents freedom from material existence and the wheel of *samsara* (life and death). The standing leg maintains the connection to life on this earth. Shiva destroys illusion and grants his devotees freedom from fear. He teaches us to distinguish between the real and unreal. Through Shiva's cosmic dance we meditate on the joy of practice and enter our own personal bliss state: *anandatandava*.

Practice

Repeat *Om Namo Shivaya,* the mantra to Shiva for overcoming fears.

Practice natarajasana consistently. Find balance between the poles of life and death.

Let your asana practice transform into sacred dance. Use music. Find the ecstasy of each breath and each gesture.

Gifts of Shiva

Risk taking, divine love, union, passion, renunciation, meditation, trance states, freedom from fear.

JR

17.

BHAIRAVI

I shall never forget Her who is the giver of
Happiness. She it is, O Mother, who, in the form of the
Moon,

Creates the world full of sounds and their meanings,
And again, by Her power in the form of the Sun, She it
is who maintains the world.
And She, again, it is who, in the form of Fire,
Destroys the whole universe at the end of the ages.

SIR JOHN WOODROFFE

18.

Now, if it so happens that you have decided to progress and if you enter the path of yoga, then a new factor intervenes. As soon as you want to progress, you immediately meet the resistance of everything that does not want to progress both in you and around you. And this resistance naturally expresses itself in all the thoughts that correspond to it.

THE MOTHER

19.

PADMASANA/LOTUS

The goddess Devi, Buddha, and others sit in padmasana, the lotus pose. As a symbol of water and fertility, the lotus flower's connection to the feminine may have originated in the pre-Vedic era of plant and animal worship or even in cultures outside of India. Female figurines from Mesopotamia, Babylonia, and Crete sit in postures similar to the lotus. Shaped from clay into spirals, they appear to be half snake/half human. One such figurine named the "snake goddess" sits in this pose of meditation.

Like the process of yoga unfolding, the lotus rises out of muddy waters to bloom in serene beauty. The blooming lotus represents the journey from darkness and confusion to clarity and light. From the shadow of dark waters the mind flowers in pure lucidity.

The lotus symbolizes and adorns the seven chakras of the yogi's subtle body, transforming the *sushumna nadi* into a garland of these life-affirming flowers. Cultivate the inner lotus through yoga practice so that the mind sits like a lotus upon water: calm and radiant.

Practice

-The hips must be open enough to sit comfortably in lotus without pain to the knees, so practice hip-opening asanas before attempting lotus.

-Sit in a sustainable position and visualize the seven chakras as lotuses.

-Visualize the space between the brows, *ajna chakra* (third eye), as a two-petaled white lotus.

-Visualize the area of the heart, *anahata chakra* (center of the sternum), as a twelve-petaled pink-and-green lotus.

-Visualize the crown of the head, *sahasrara chakra*, as the shining bright, thousand-petaled lotus opening to liberation.

JR

20.

The mind is like the wind and the body is like the sand; if you want to know how the wind is blowing, you can look at the sand.

BONNIE BAINBRIDGE-COHEN

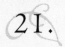

21.

But as to whether one really needs his own teacher or not generally, books can be the teacher. When one Tibetan lama was about to die, he said to his disciple, "Now you should no longer rely on a human teacher, but you should rely on books to be your teacher." I think that's very wise. Without investigation and without knowing a person properly you may hurriedly take someone as your guru or teacher, and there is too much involved in guru devotion or guru yoga. So it could land you in trouble. The thorough investigation of a teacher is very, very important.

THE DALAI LAMA

22.

INTEGRATION

Like water being wrung from a cloth, the process of yoga drains us of past conditioning. Negative *samskara* and the pain of repetition are replaced with more positive habits. Yoga unpacks us particle by particle, cell by cell. Its integrative force pulls us together again. Like fearless explorers, we dive into the body unwinding the knots that bind. We then begin to live in tune with the energies of the subtle body, or at least we can catch moments of this.

JR

23.

Consider a lake. Does the water touch the banks only on one side and not on the other, or does it touch the banks equally everywhere? When you are performing an asana, your consciousness, like the waters of a lake, should touch the frontiers of the body everywhere. Where, then, is there room for thoughts to arise? How can there be a thought arising when you are doing a perfect asana—when your intelligence has spread through your whole body?

B. K. S. IYENGAR

24.

Yoga is a generic name for any discipline by which one attempts to pass out of the limits of ones's ordinary mental consciousness into a greater spiritual consciousness.

SRI AUROBINDO

25.

Q: Yoga means to join. Is it like many grains together?
A: It's like sugar and water or salt and water.

SRI T. KRISHNAMACHARYA

26.

YOUR YOGA

Integration through yoga requires intelligence, humility, and humor. A good guide and a willingness to live and feel fully will help you on your journey. As you progress, you will learn to craft your practice like an artist.

The medium that you work with is not paint or clay but your own body/mind. Over time you will no longer be satisfied with imitation but will find your soul's unique expression, and your example will inspire others.

Practice

Commit to a daily home practice. Twenty minutes a day is a good starting place.

JR

27.

Foremost amongst devotees are those who are one-
    pointed.
Conversing with each other with voices choking, hairs
    standing on end, and tears in their eyes, they purify
    their communities and the earth. . . .
Among them, distinctions of ancestry, intellect, appear-
    ance, class, wealth, occupation, and
    other social realities are irrelevant.

BHAKTI NARADA SUTRAS

28.

There was never born neither the mind nor the objects perceived by the mind. Those who perceive such births may as well try to perceive the footprints of the birds in the sky.

MANDUKYA UPANISHAD

29.

STASIS AND CHANGE

Physical postures are potent tools for both stasis and change, for working with pleasure, pain, and fear. For example, the feelings generated from back-bending postures can result in a kind of euphoria, yet the prospect of moving deeper into the back bend may bring up intense fear and dread. Finding the axis between moving forward (or backward) more deeply into a pose and backing off is the work of yoga and the perfect metaphor for negotiating intimacy with ourselves and with others. These choice points require attention and will transport yoga practice from a simple body/culture activity into the true workings of personal transformation.

JR

30.

Meditation is your intrinsic nature
—it is you.
It has nothing to do
with your doings:
you cannot have it,
you cannot not have it,
it cannot be possessed,
it is not a thing, it is you.

OSHO

31.

If the dream says something is wrong with your body,
   check.
Long before you do, your body knows when something is
   wrong.

MARION WOODMAN

32.

DOLPHIN POSE

Dolphins are the intelligence of the sea. Through the practice of the dolphin pose not only do we gain sea mammal wisdom but we also empathize with their plight. Every day more and more sea mammals and creatures of all kinds lose habitat due to human interference in the ocean, forests, and mountains. The ancients practiced the animal poses as a way to reflect and honor the natural world to which we each belong.

The next time that you practice dolphin or tree (or any of the animal poses), ally your mind with these creatures and meditate on healing the oceans and forests. Make your practice a prayer for peace (ahimsa) for all living creatures. Cultivate stewardship of the land and sea.

JR

33.

Will you never have done? (Pause) Will you never have done . . . revolving it all? (Pause) It? (Pause) It all. (Pause) In your poor mind. (Pause) It all. (Pause) It all.

SAMUEL BECKETT

34.

. . . everyone was telling me to continue practicing, you see. But I wasn't satisfied. Because my experience was that the practices left by themselves. I loved them. I was puzzled because I could not do them. I could not sit. So I went to my master to solve this problem. I went on my Saturday holiday. I said, "I have been practicing for eighteen years, always meditating. I woke up and didn't want to sit. I am confused about what to do." Then he asked me,

"How did you come from Madras to Tiruvannamalai?"

I answered, "By train."

"And from the railway station to the ashram?"

"By horse cart."

"Where are these?"

I said I had left them at their stations. He said, "The means brought you to a place and you rejected the means. They left you. Means will bring you, introduce you, and turn back. You can't keep sitting on the train when the ride is over. The work of the practice has taken you to your destination; now get out at the station. The work of the practice is over now and you have to face yourself—a very pleasing situation."

ELI JAXON-BEAR

SATSANG WITH H. W. L. POONJA

35.

The door to the soul lies in the breath.

JR

36.

A good group is better than a spectacular group.
When leaders become superstars, the teacher outshines
the teaching.

LAO TZU'S TAO TE CHING, ADAPTED FOR A NEW AGE

37.

Ahimsa covers thought as well as action. Patanjali recommends that your yoga practice be based on the determination to avoid not just harmful actions, but even thoughts that could harm another being. Non-harming is essential to the yogi because it creates good karma—not only for the person or animal that is not harmed, but for the yogi who has refrained from causing harm . . .

Compassion is an essential ingredient of ahimsa. Through compassion you begin to see yourself in other beings. This helps you refrain from causing harm to them. Developing compassion does something else, however, which is of special interest to the yogi. It trains the mind to see outer differences of form. You begin to catch the essence of other beings which is happiness.

SHARON GANNON AND DAVID LIFE

38.

Go on saying, "I am free." Never mind if the next moment delusion comes and says, "I am bound." Dehypnotize the whole thing.

SWAMI VIVEKANANDA

39.

VAYU

Five winds, known as *vayus*, or pranas, regulate the energy in the body. These *vayus* are associated with consciousness, breath, and the practice of pranayama. The two primary *vayus* are known as prana and *apana*. Prana ascends the breath energy with inhalation, while *apana* directs the flow of energy downward and connects us to the earth with exhalation. The incoming breath, associated with the navel and heart regions, promotes mental clarity while too much of this prana can cause spaciness and dissociation. The *apana* action of digestive elimination, located in the lower half of the trunk, makes us feel strong like the root of a tree or plant. In excess, this force creates a sense of heaviness like trying to walk through mud. A third *vayu* known as *vyana* circulates the breath throughout the body's periphery into the limbs. The mingling of *apana* with prana brings about yoga integration and states of higher consciousness and well-being.

Grounding Practice

-Stand with legs two feet apart and slightly turned out. Inhale and draw the hands upward toward the sky. Exhale and bend the knees into a half squat while drawing the hands down toward the earth. Repeat ten times. You may introduce the sound *lam* (for the root chakra).

-When exhaling focus on letting go.

-When inhaling focus on abundance and energy.

JR

40.

POSTERITY

Armed with their rules and precepts, many condemn my
    verses.
I don't write for them,
but for that soul, twin to mine, who will be born
    tomorrow.
Time is long and the world wide.

BHAVABHUTI

41.

Suddenly, with a roar like that of a waterfall, I felt a stream of
liquid light entering my brain through the spinal cord. Entirely
unprepared for such a development, I was completely taken by
surprise; but regaining my self-control, keeping my mind on the

point of concentration. The illumination grew brighter and brighter, the roaring louder, I experienced a rocking sensation and then felt myself slipping out of my body, entirely enveloped in a halo of light. It is impossible to describe the experience accurately. I felt the point of consciousness that was myself growing wider surrounded by waves of light. It grew wider and wider, spreading outward while the body, normally the immediate object of its perception, appeared to have receded into the distance until I became entirely unconscious of it. I was now all consciousness without any outline, without any idea of corporeal appendage, without any feeling or sensation coming from the senses, immersed in a sea of light simultaneously conscious and aware at every point, spread out, as it were, in all directions without any barrier or material obstruction. I was no longer myself, or to be more accurate, no longer as I knew myself to be, a small point of awareness confined to a body, but instead was a vast circle of consciousness in which the body was but a point, bathed in light and in a state of exaltation and happiness impossible to describe.

GOPI KRISHNA

42.

BHAKTI YOGA

Perhaps the most direct route to yoga, bhakti is the yoga of devotion and the yoga of love. Surrendering to the divine and serving God consumes the bhakta (one who practices bhakti). On this path of love, all efforts are offered up as prayer. All work, relationships, and activities are seen as part of the sacred play (*lila*) of life.

The bhakta finds expression in music, poetry, and dance. The intense longing for the divine finds its expression through these devotional practices. The sacred singing of *bhajan* and *raga* brings the devotee closer to a divine presence and is embraced with abandon. The Indian mystics Mirabai and Kabir and the Persian poet Rumi exemplify the practice of bhakti.

Practice

Every aspect of our yoga practice from asana to song and from cooking to meditation can be embodied as bhakti. This attitude, cultivated through yoga and shared with others through our daily reverie of prayer, song, and practice, makes the heart sing.

-Sing, chant, or hum during asana practice and while
  performing daily tasks.
-Create an altar with inspiring images.
-Create a mental image of someone you care for who
  might need healing as part of your bhakti meditation.

JR

43.

It's like when we begin to see the work that is to be done, and we
go to an ashram or a monastery, or we hang out with satsang. We
surround ourselves with a community of beings who think the
way we think. And then none of the stuff, the really hairy stuff
inside ourselves, comes up. It all gets pushed underground. We
can sit in a temple or a cave in India and get so holy, so clear and
radiant, the light is pouring out of us. But when we come out of
that cave, when we leave that supportive structure which worked
with our strengths but seldom confronted us with our weak-
nesses, our old habit patterns tend to reappear, and we come back
into the same old games, the games we were sure we had finished
with. Because there were uncooked seeds, seeds of desires that

sprout again the minute they are stimulated. We can stay in very holy places, and the seeds sit there dormant and uncooked.

RAM DASS

44.

This Soul of mine within the heart is smaller than a grain of rice, or a barley-corn, or a mustard seed, or a grain of millet, or the kernel of a grain of millet; this Soul of mine within the heart is greater than the earth, greater than the atmosphere, greater than the sky, greater than these worlds. Containing all works, containing all desires, containing all odors, containing all tastes, encompassing the whole world, the unspeaking the unconcerned—this soul of mine within the heart, this is Brahman.

CHANDOGYA UPANISHAD

45.

From the conversation and the books of some of my friends I have been almost led to conclude that happiness in the modern world has become an impossibility. I find, however, that this view tends to be dissipated by introspection, foreign travel, and the conversation of my gardener.

BERTRAND RUSSELL

46.

INTENTION

Setting an intention for each yoga session increases mental focus and creates a vibrant practice. Intentions can be general or specific, abstract or concrete. Some examples: "My intention today is to make peace with myself (or a specific other) both in my practice and throughout this day" or "Let me complete one hour of yoga practice." You might think of them as little prayers sprinkled over your practice time.

JR

In the secret cave of the heart, two are seated by life's
    fountain.
The separate ego drinks of the sweet and bitter stuff,
Liking the sweet, disliking the bitter,
While the supreme Self drinks sweet and bitter
Neither liking this nor disliking that.
The ego gropes in darkness, while the Self lives in light.

KATHA UPANISHAD

48.

If we are to reach real peace in this world and if we are to carry on a real war against war, we shall have to begin with children; and if they will grow up in their natural innocence, we won't have to struggle; we won't have to pass fruitless idle resolutions, but we shall go from love to love and peace to peace, until at last all the corners of the world are covered with that peace and love for which consciously or unconsciously the whole world is hungering.

GANDHI

49.

Rising, sitting down, walking, in fact any gesture taken up by the body is called an asana. It corresponds to the rhythm and the vibration of body and mind at any particular moment. Some aspirants can meditate only if seated in the pose indicated by the Guru or formulated in the shastras scriptures and not otherwise.

This is the way to proficiency in meditation. On the other hand, someone may begin his practice while sitting in any ordinary position; nevertheless, as soon as the state of *japa*, repetition of a mantra or dhyana, concentration has been reached, the body will spontaneously take up the most appropriate position. As one's meditation grows increasingly intense, the postures correspondingly gain in perfection. When a little air is pumped into a tyre, the tyre will be flabby; but when it is filled to capacity, it remains completely stable in its own natural shape. Likewise when real meditation has been attained, the body feels light and free, and on rising after meditation there is no fatigue of any kind, no pain, numbness or stiffness in one's limbs.

SRI ANANDAMAYI MA

50.

If something is boring after two minutes, try it for four. If it is still boring try it for eight, sixteen, thirty-two, and so on. Eventually one discovers that it's not boring at all but very interesting.

JOHN CAGE

51.

RESTLESS MIND

Yoga brings us face-to-face with the restless mind. In the beginning of yoga practice the mind moves toward peace, toward more distraction, or toward a fluctuation between these two.

Practice
Let your yoga *sadhana* bring fresh perspective to the various dilemmas that you may encounter in your life. First, step apart from

your personal problems and practice. Notice what comes up. Is your mind racing during practice? Can you use the breath to steady and soften the thinking—mind? The process of yoga itself can shift the grooves in the mind as they drop away like autumn leaves from a tree. Then you begin to access *buddhi* (discriminating intelligence). Note how you feel before and after your practice. Have your habitual concerns eased up?

JR

52.

Hafiz our great and wonderful poet of Persia, says: Many say that life entered the human body by the help of music, but the truth is that life itself is music. I should like to tell you what made him say this:

There exists in the East a legend which relates that God made a statue of clay in His own image, and asked the soul to enter into it. But the soul refused to enter into this prison, for its nature is to fly about freely, and not be limited and bound to any sort of captivity. The soul did not wish in the least to enter this prison. Then God asked the

angels to play their music and, as the angels played, the soul was
moved to ecstasy. Through that ecstasy—in order to make this music
more clear to itself—it entered this body.

HAZRAT INAYAT KHAN

The earliest primordial images of the Earth Mother glorified a fecundating principle that held within itself the secrets of birth and death . . . Through the centuries having shed her aniconic presence, the primeval Mother was manifest, evolving from hieroglyph to plant, to animal and finally to the human Shakti with a thousand names and forms. Potent with energy, holding within her the essence of her earlier incarnation, she had the capacity to heal and transform. For the essences of her earlier incarnations had been absorbed into herself; the triangle and hieroglyph rested on her heart or her generative organs, the vegetal side of her nature was manifest in the plants she held in her hands, her animal incarnations were transformed into her vehicle . . . In her final manifestation she was Durga, the goddess of elemental form, holder of all life, brighter than a thousand suns.

PUPUL JAYAKAR

54.

This body Arjuna, is called the field.
He who knows this is called the knower of the field.

BHAGAVAD GITA 13:1

55.

What is essential here is the presence of the spirit of dialogue, which is in short, the ability to hold many points of view in suspension, along with a primary interest in the creation of common meaning.

DAVID BOHM

56.

The beginning: something not to be found in nature. The first distinct image was that of Vishnu drifting on the waters, his head reclined on Sesa. In the image that precedes all others, Vishnu was already resting on the past. The first world was always at least the second, always concealed within it another that had come before. . . . Sesa was also *sefa*, the "residue" one meets every day: food leftovers, remainders in division, the remnants of our actions, which are still there even when the fruit of the action has been consumed, on the earth and in the sky. From that residue new life develops. The new is an old, old lump, which refuses to dissolve.

ROBERTO CALASSO

57.

PAUSE

Rest in the pause between breaths.
Pause in the rest between thoughts.

Bask in the space between words.
Stop in the stillness between time.

JR

58.

HANUMANASANA—MONKEY
GOD'S POSE

An incarnation of Lord Shiva and a devoted servant to the god
Ram, the monkey god, Hanuman, is also the son of Vayu, god of
the wind. He represents courage, strength, and power and assumes the form of a monkey in which to do his divine work.

When the demon Ravanna kidnaps the goddess Sita (keeping her from her husband, Ram) Hanuman leaps across the sea to Lanka where Sita is held captive. Hanuman's lucidity and pure heart lead him to Sita so that she may be liberated. He rescues her and thus serves his lord with success and devotion.

Hanuman's leap, similar to a ballet split, reflects his ability to extend himself selflessly. The gift of this deeply stretched pose breaks through the barriers that block pure perception to liberate us, just as Sita, too, becomes free.

Practice
The practice of hanumanasana helps us to explore our edges.

-Where do you hold back in your practice?
-Where could you go deeper or further?

JR

59.

Another important dimension in yoga is learning how to "play the edge." The body has edges that mark its limits in stretch, strength, endurance, and balance. The flexibility edge can be used to illustrate this. In each posture, at any given time, there is a limit to stretch that I call the final or "maximum edge." This edge has a feeling of intensity, and is right before pain, but it is not pain itself. The edge moves from day to day and from breath to breath. It does not always move forward; sometimes it retreats. Part of learning how to do yoga is learning how to surrender to this edge, so that when it changes you move with the change. It is psychologically easier to move forward than to back off. But it's as important to learn to move back if your edge closes, as it is to learn to move forward slowly as the body opens.

JOEL KRAMER

60.

When the pupil is ready the teacher appears.

YOGI RAMACHARAKA

61.

It is possible to say that there are certain distinctions between yoga and Hinduism. There are also fundamental differences between yoga and Vedanta. And if at all we can link them, it is as follows: yoga is the means towards Vedanta for those who are interested. Vedanta involves a lot of inquiry and reflection, and also demands the development of bhakti, and, both for the mind and for the individual, yoga is the means towards bhakti.

T. K. V. DESIKACHAR

62.

PRAYER FOR WHOLENESS—
PEACE INVOCATION

OM Purnamadah, purnamidam purnat
Purnamadachyate
Purnasya purnamadaya
Purnameveva shishate
Om Shanti! Shanti! Shanti!

OM! That is whole. This is whole;
From the whole the whole becomes manifest.
From the whole when the whole is negated,
what remains is again the whole
Om Peace! Peace! Peace!

ISAVASYA UPANISHAD

63.

If you find a good solution and become attached to it, the solution may become your next problem.

ROBERT ANTHONY

64.

Perhaps I was sleeping when I came into the one realization that continues to sustain me: "If you know who walks beside you, you can never be afraid!" I wish I knew the exact moment and time it happened because I would have had a party. I now believe it was in that instant that my soul opened up and the spirit of the Divine entered my life. I have met hundreds of thousands of people I recognize from my own experiences to be utterly insane. It is not the kind of insanity that will get you tossed into the looney bin. It is a kind of insanity that keeps you in a struggle for control of your life and everyone in it. The kind of insanity we are talking about here is a kind that keeps you pushing yourself, striving to do more, be better, and get ahead. Unfortunately, because you are insane, when you get ahead, when you are better, when you get more, it is still not enough. The insanity that plagues more than half of the adult population of most countries is a kind that makes fully capable, able-bodied people stay in jobs in which they are miserable. These insane people stay in relationships where they cheat or are cheated on. They remain in situations of all kinds where they are abused, neglected, demeaned, overlooked, and, in many ways I cannot enumerate, otherwise dehumanized. The insanity I am identifying here is the kind that makes you forget who walks beside you and who lives within you and that, as a result of this loss of memory, shuts down your soul.

IYANLA VANZANT

65.

We do not live our life out and full; we do not fill all our pores with our blood; we do not inspire and expire fully and entirely enough, so that the wave, the comber, of each inspiration shall break upon our extremest shores, rolling till it meets the sand which bounds us, and the sound of the surf comes back to us. Might not a bellows assist us to breathe? That our breathing should create a wind in a calm day! We live but a fraction of our life. Why do we not let on the flood, raise the gates, and set all our wheels in motion? He that hath ears to hear, let him hear.

HENRY DAVID THOREAU

66.

What is the witness soul?

It is the soul entering into a state in which it observes without acting. A witness is one who *looks* at what is *done*, but does not act himself. So when the soul is in a state in which it does not participate in the action, does not act through Nature, simply draws back and observes, it becomes the witness soul. . . .

THE MOTHER

67.

ODE TO SHIVA

In this body there exists a cave,
A dwelling place
Where Lord Shiva and I meet daily for yoga practice:

You remind me to sit for a thousand years.
To leave all action and act as witness to myself in stillness.
All the creatures of the forest gather round,
Alone not alone.
When the sitting is too much for my mortal body I get up
    to dance the dance of the universe.

Sometimes I rage and burn as a fire lights under my pounding feet.
This yoga is not quiet as the world pulses to a god's pace.

But the dance must finish and I will leave this body and we
   will sit again You and I, in the forest under the
   stars and the moon.

JR

68.

When the movement in the direction of becoming something other than what you are isn't there anymore, you are not in conflict with yourself.

U. G. KRISHNAMURTI

In the first stage, when the heart chakra is pierced, we hear tinkling sounds like jewels in the space of the heart in the center of the body. As soon as these sounds become audible in the (interior) void, the yogi becomes godlike, radiant, healthy, and fragrant. His heart becomes the void.

HATHA YOGA PRADIPIKA

Rise, awake! having obtained your boons, understand them! The sharp edge of a razor is difficult to pass over; thus the wise say the path (to the Self) is hard.

KATHA UPANISHAD

71.

From where does sound manifest? From where has it come? Where does it go? It merges into the ether, the *sunyatta*, and then it reemerges. Whether we are in the sound, or the sound is in us, it is always a mystery. Even when we are not striking up any sound, does the unstruck sound not emanate through us, in spite of us? The ocean of sound is composed of that struck and unstruck sound, all rolled into One. And we are a part of that. The drop is in the ocean. But the drop in the ocean can say, yes I am ocean.

Are we sound?

We are sound. Aren't we? When we are in control of sound, then we *are* sound. And that sound is just like when you hold a set of scales. On one side you keep the weight, on the other you keep the goods. So sound is balanced with silence. You cannot be fully aware of the beauty of this sound unless you have tasted silence.

SRI KARUNAMAYEE

72.

There is no virtue or vice for me, no pleasure or pain
   for me,
no incantations, no pilgrimage, no scriptures, no sacrifi-
   cial rites
are there for me! I am neither the enjoyer nor the enjoyed
   nor the enjoyment. I am
Auspiciousness (Siva) , Consciousness and Bliss. Verily I
   am the blissful form of the
Auspiciousness (Siva).

SRI SHANKARACHARYA

73.

COMFORT ZONE

We must stay attuned to how we approach yoga, otherwise we run the risk of staying firmly in our comfort zones. When we become attached to certain approaches—or even to certain "styles"—of yoga, we will find we cannot operate outside these domains. We fall into a trance and work under the illusion that change is happening, when actually the yoga is serving to reinforce our habits. We keep swimming, but never leave familiar waters.

JR

74.

THE STAIRWAY OF EXISTENCE

We are not
In pursuit of formalities

Or fake religious
Laws,

For through the stairway of existence
We have come to God's Door.

We are
People who need to love, because
Love is the soul's life,
Love is simply creation's greatest joy.
Through
The stairway of existence,
O, Through the stairway of existence, Hafiz
Have
You now come,
Have we all now come to
The Beloved's
Door.

HAFIZ

75.

So let us move into the next millennium with hope, for without it all we can do is eat and drink the last of our resources as we watch our planet slowly die. Instead, let us have faith in ourselves, in our intellect, in our staunch spirit. Let us develop respect for all living things. Let us try to replace impatience and intolerance with understanding and compassion. And love.

JANE GOODALL

76.

PASCHIMOTTANASANA

Seated-Forward Bend: Head-to-Foot Pose
Sit bones connect to the earth. Inhaling, I raise my arms. Exhaling, I move my torso forward and down over my legs. I stretch my spine awakening to the new day before me. I leave the past be-

hind. My exhale extends as I release what binds me to pain or expectation. This intensely stretched seat pulls me into moments of
deep letting go.

Faithful practice of this pose brings great results. I take refuge
here, gazing at the front of my legs, or touching my head all the
way down. Not much is down here on the ground and everything
is down here: the Self and a daily encounter with myself.

JR

Asato Ma sad gamaya
Tamaso Ma jyotir gamaya
Mrityur Ma amritam gamaya

Mother!
From untruth, lead me to truth,
From darkness, lead me toward the light,
From death, lead me to eternal life.

BRIHADARANYAKA UPANISHAD

The demons aren't the noise. They are our aversion to the noise. . . .

When you can accept discomfort, doing so allows a balance of mind. That surrender, that letting go of wanting anything to be other than it is right in the moment, is what frees us from hell.

STEPHEN LEVINE

There is nothing in a caterpillar that tells you it's going to be a butterfly.

RICHARD BUCKMINSTER FULLER

80.

Witnessing is spontaneous and in the present moment. Therefore any thought which arises gets cut off. It may come up again but again when it is witnessed it gets cut off. Each time it arises it gets cut off. As Ramana Maharshi said, "It is like an uninvited guest who, when ignored, gradually stops coming."

RAMESH BALSEKAR

81.

That wise Yogi who daily drinks the ambrosial air, according to the rules, destroys fatigue, burning (fever) decay and old age, and injuries.

Pointing the tongue upward, when the Yogi can drink the nectar flowing from the moon (situated between the two eyebrows) within a month he would certainly conquer death.

When having firmly closed the glottis by the proper yogic method, and contemplating on the goddess Kundalini, he drinks (the moon fluid of immortality), he becomes a sage or a poet within six months.

SIVA SAMHITA

82.

People can learn movement in a variety of ways. They are not necessarily enabled to feel it when they do so. It is the concrete, specific awareness of one's own act of moving which is so satisfying. The physical culture courses of which our friend spoke, work with the body as object not as subject, and while a general release takes place, there is no corresponding experience of the personal identity, its quality and its movement. This seems to mean that something more is needed than simply body mechanics, that the feelings hidden in the body, the source of all its movement, must be involved. People in general are not very interested in abdominal muscles, the diaphragm, the shoulder girdle and the pelvis, but they care deeply about the world in which they must find a way to live and about themselves who must do the living.

MARY STARKS WHITEHOUSE

83.

GANGA'S TALE

Sometime prior to written history, drought scorched the land now called India. King Bharaivi implored the great goddess Ganga, also known as "the wild one," to intervene. He stood on one leg in vriksasana (tree pose) for many months doing penance to save the earth.

"Shower your waters upon us, dear one," he prayed.

The wild and playful Ganga, hearing his call, reveled in the chance to flood the earth with abandon. With much delight and filled with immense *shakti*, Ganga swirled like a great tidal wave and unleashed her powerful waters. Lord Shiva, hearing of this deluge, rushed to catch Ganga upon his head of matted hair.

Holding her there lessened the impact of her descent to earth and consummated the Shiva/Shakti union. Masculine and feminine energies mingled in this divine embrace, and the two great gods became eternal playmates. As rivers great and small flowed down from Shiva's head, including the great Ganges herself, the deadly drought was averted.

Look closely and you may spot Ganga caught in the bun atop Shiva's head as she replenishes the rivers and the lakes. To this day, the Ganges is honored as one of India's most holy places. For Hindus, bathing in her waters before dying ensures a safe journey to the next life.

JR

84.

There is a vitality, a life force, an energy, a quickening that is translated through you into action, and because there is only one of you in all time. This expression is unique. And if you block it, it will never exist through any other medium and will be lost.

MARTHA GRAHAM

85.

MIRROR

Yoga acts as a mirror. Each breath, each movement, reflects to us who we are and how we are moment to moment. We look into the mirror of yoga and see the places that need support and the places that need to open. The postures teach us about ourselves, markers on the map of the soul. They bless us with immediate feedback. As we move deeper into the physical and mystical teachings, we become intrepid explorers mining the terrain of body, mind, and soul.

JR

Truth is a pathless land, and you cannot approach it by any path whatsoever, by any religion, by any sect. Truth, being limitless, unconditioned, unapproachable by any path whatsoever, cannot be organized; nor should any organization be formed to lead or to coerce people along any particular path.

J. KRISHNAMURTI

87.

CHAKRA SYSTEM

Chakras make up an important part of the Hatha Yoga and Tantra Yoga systems and permeate the subtle body of the yogi. Depicted as lotus flowers, these energy centers, or wheels, adorn the central axis known as the *sushumna nadi*. Each chakra has a location near physical parts of the body (i.e., throat, heart) but should not be confused with the actual physical places themselves. Instead, they bridge the gross and etheric planes and represent the inner or alchemical body of the yoga practitioner. The ability to sense these different centers can be cultivated through asana, pranayama, meditation, and sound. Chakra work opens us up to the vast field of the inner body and facilitates intense awareness and healing.

JR

88.

When I jumped up like a madman and seized [a sword], suddenly the blessed Mother revealed herself. The buildings with their different parts, the temple, and everything vanished from my sight, leaving no trace whatsoever, and in their stead I saw a limitless, infinite, effulgent Ocean of Consciousness. As far as the eye could see, the shining billows were madly rushing at me from all sides with a terrific noise, to swallow me up. I was caught in the rush and collapsed, unconscious. . . . Within me there was a steady flow of undiluted bliss, altogether new, and I felt the presence of the Divine Mother.

SRI RAMAKRISHNA

89.

More than fifteen years later a highly cultivated Indian visited me, a friend of Gandhi's, and we talked about Indian education—in particular, about the relationship between guru and *chela*. I hesitantly asked him whether he could tell me anything about the person and character of his own guru, whereupon he replied in a matter-of-fact tone, "Oh yes, he was Shankaracharya."

"You don't mean the commentator on the Vedas who died centuries ago?" I asked.

"Yes, I mean him," he said, to my amazement.

"Then you are referring to a spirit?" I asked.

"Of course it was his spirit," he agreed.

"There are ghostly gurus too," he added. "Most people have living gurus. But there are always some who have a spirit for teacher."

C. G. JUNG

90.

Sometimes, when resistance ceases, the pain simply goes away or dwindles to an easily tolerable ache. At other times it remains, but the absence of any resistance brings about a way of feeling pain so unfamiliar as to be hard to describe. The pain is no longer *problematic*. I feel it, but there is no urge to get rid of it, for I have discovered that pain and the effort to be separate from it are the same thing. Wanting to get out of pain *is* the pain; it is not the "reaction" of an "I" distinct from the pain. When you discover this, the desire to escape "merges" into the pain itself and *vanishes*.

ALAN WATTS

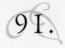

91.

BREATH BEFORE DAWN

As I wake this morning I begin to visualize my yoga practice. I make tea and gaze outside my window. All the while in the background I wonder what is holding me back from the mat or from meditation or from sound. I know that all roads lead to my practice, no matter how many small tasks I put in front of me. I see these roadblocks and wonder why resistance crops up around something so worthwhile. My mind trips me up. The transition from sleep to practice is not always the way I intend. The judgments start to creep in before I remind myself to let go and accept where I am. I remember that yoga practice is a joy and a privilege and something that I choose. So I plunge ahead and watch the resistance burn up in the warmth of my body moving through space and the sound of my breath before dawn.

JR

92.

Love is manifest where there is an able vessel.

BHAKTI NARADA SUTRAS

93.

I am the ritual and the worship, the medicine and the mantra,
the butter burnt in the fire,
and I am the flames that consume it.

I am the father of the universe
and its mother, essence and goal of all knowledge, the
    refiner, the sacred Om, and the threefold Vedas.

I am the beginning and the end, origin and dissolution,
    refuge, home, true lover, womb, and imperishable seed.

BHAGAVAD GITA 9:16

94.

The Los Angelization of yoga is not unlike an organic fruit wrapped in twenty thousand layers of nonrecyclable, nonbiodegradable packages, not unlike a sports utility vehicle. We are mobile, we have tasted the pure thing, we have ways to preserve and to run from it. To own it and contain it. To overdo it.

The Americanization of yoga includes strain. A higher rate of injury than from yoga practiced in Asian countries. Emphasis on postures only. Competition. Merchandise: mats, pillows, eye bags, blankets, blocks, ropes, tanks, shorts, T-shirts, J. Crew yoga clothes. Overkill. The terms *power yoga, yoga workout.* Water bottles. Office yoga . . . Yoga becomes something we must own. In our decade, yoga is something to market. To market, to market, the latest way to forget.

REETIKA VAZIRANI

95.

There are two ways of spreading light: to be the candle or the
mirror that reflects it.

EDITH WHARTON

96.

THE PRACTICE

Today, I wake. Sort of. Roll out of bed. Make tea.
Awaiting the moment of practice.
It never comes.
I notice this moment of never coming practice.
I notice.

JR

97.

When the highest purpose of life is achieved, the three basic qualities do not excite responses in the mind. That is freedom. In other words, the Perceiver is no longer colored by the mind.

YOGA SUTRA OF PATANJALI IV:34

98.

Why indeed must "God" be a noun? Why not a verb—the most active and dynamic of all?

MARY DALY

99.

SALAMBA SIRSASANA: THE PROMISE OF THE POSE

On this soft blanket of grass,
My crown links with earth, my feet with sky.
Balanced between darkness and light, I enter the earth's
    round body.
I sense the velocity of speed and light.
Wobbling, gravity tugs at me.
How quickly we spin through this galaxy. How relative my
    place within it.

Perched on my head, my perspective as to what is up shifts
    and
all confusion and clutter escape in the promise of the pose.

Practice

Assume a child's mind and practice falling out of the headstand on soft grass. Don't waste your fall. Falls are useful. They teach us about balance. Find out what happened to pull you down. Be your own mirror or get your teacher to help you. Enjoy the ride.

JR

100.

Anyone who actively practices yoga, be he young, old, or even very old, sickly or weak, can become a *siddha*.

HATHA YOGA PRADIPIKA

101.

. . . you carry in yourself all the obstacles necessary to make your realization perfect. Always you will see that within you the shadow and the light are equal: you have an ability, you have also the negation of this ability. But if you discover a very black hole, a thick shadow, be sure there is somewhere in you a great light. It is up to you to know how to use the one to realize the other.

THE MOTHER

102.

YOGINI

Female yoga practitioners, known as yoginis, have practiced yoga for millennia. Archaeological evidence points to the practice of yoga as part of ancient fertility rites. Medieval miniature paintings depict yoginis wandering the forest, playing music, and as ascetics sitting with disciples and animals in meditation. These female mystics played an important role in the spiritual life of the community and wielded a certain amount of authority. The mystical poet Mirabai devoted her life to composing verse and music as an offering to the divine. Today, well-known female gurus like Ammachi in South India and Guru Mai continue the tradition of women as spiritual leaders and mystics.

In Tantric ritual, yoginis played a pivotal role as holders of *shakti.* The famous yogini temples in Orissa show the majesty of the female body in all its guises and strengths. These temples are testament to the intensity with which spiritual knowledge of the divine feminine was honored and pursued by those both within and outside orthodox Brahmanic culture. The yogini lineage has spread throughout the world—evident in the millions of modern women devoted to the daily practice of yoga.

Practice
Whether male or female (yogi or yogini), find a way to honor the divine feminine within. This force creates all birth and all life. Honor your own *shakti*.

JR

I03.

I stood on the path,
no one saw my pain,
A guru passed,
he gave me medicine,
every pore found peace . . .

MIRABAI

104.

Mama may have,
Papa may have,
But God bless the child that's got his own,
That's got his own.

"GOD BLESS THE CHILD," GOSPEL SONG

105.

The practice of Yoga brings us face-to-face with the extraordinary complexity of our own being, the stimulating but also embarrassing multiplicity of our personality, the rich endless confusion of Nature. To the ordinary man who lives upon his own waking surface, ignorant of the self's depths and vastness behind the veil, his psychological existence is fairly simple. . . .

For our real self is not the individual mental being, that is only a figure, an appearance; our real self is cosmic, infinite, it is stop. The student pours. The master says nothing. The cup begins to overflow, and still the master remains silent. Upset, the student exclaims:

"Master, look at this tea cup! It is full and overflowing!"

The master replies: "Yes. Just as your mind is already full. None of this teaching will be of benefit until you empty your cup."

The disciple learned the first lesson of spiritual teaching: to be empty of preconceptions and receptive to new knowledge.

JR

107.

Various religions, Bibles, Vedas, dogmas—are all just tubs for the little plant; but it must get out of the tub.

SWAMI VIVEKANANDA

one with all existence and the inhabitant of all existence. The self behind our mind, life and body is the same as the self behind the mind, life and body of all our fellow-beings, and if we come to possess it, we shall naturally, when we turn to look out again upon them, tend to become one with them in the common basis of our consciousness.

SRI AUROBINDO

106.

FULL CUP, EMPTY CUP

A popular Zen story tells of a disciple who embarks on a journey in search of a master teacher. When the teacher appears, the student becomes excited and begins asking questions hoping to gain wisdom. Eager to have her questions answered, the student persists but the teacher refuses to rectly. Instead she requests that the student pour The teacher tells the student to keep pouring unt

108.

Knowing all objects to be impermanent
let not their contact bind you
resolve again and again to be aware of the Self that is
permanent.

SRI T. KRISHNAMACHARYA

109.

My teacher's pure perception of me, just as I am, helped me to
connect more completely to who I am. In the mirror of the awakened teacher's clear seeing, I could better know my higher sense
and my true inner nature. I had a distorted picture of myself, and
perhaps you have one of yourself. These invaluable Dharma teachings encouraged me to know that it is possible for everyone—not
just a guru or a monk, and not just the Buddha—but me and you
too—to connect to the Buddha within. The authentic Buddha is

beyond time and place, beyond gender, beyond form or nationality. You carry a Buddha with you right now, in your heart.

LAMA SURYA DAS

110.

In the Lord of Yoga is the incomparable seed of omniscience. Being unconditioned by time, it is the teacher of even the ancient teachers. Its sound is the reverberating syllable AUM. Repetition of this syllable reveals its meaning.

YOGA SUTRA OF PATANJALI I:25–28

III.

... My Love,
he is here
inside
   He does not leave,
He doesn't
Need to arrive.

MIRABAI

II2.

THE DOG DAYS OF YOGA—OR
WHAT TO DO WHEN THE YOGA
MUSE IS ALL DRIED UP

Some days we don't feel up to it. We tire of our regular class or
practice, and feel exhausted, sick, hungry, or depressed. Maybe

we're too busy, too stressed or preoccupied. We make excuses: "Can't afford it." "There's no parking." "It's too hot." "It's too cold." "It's raining." I know. I've been there. If you lack the motivation to do your usual practice, change it. Maybe your practice is so full of asana that what you need is to sit or chant or sing. Find a restorative pose. Adapt your practice to your needs.

JR

113.

At that moment, the universe appeared to disclose its hidden reality: it was in perpetual transformation. What was apparently stable melted away into the moving: what was apparently finite sank into the infinite. There was no fixed, final state. And is that not the real truth, since all living things are but condensation of the breath?

FRANÇOIS CHENG

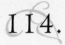

114.

Those who know this truth, whose consciousness is unified, think always, "I am not the doer." While seeing or hearing, touching or smelling; eating, moving about, or sleeping; breathing or speaking, letting go or holding on, even opening or closing the eyes, they understand that these are only the movements of the senses among sense objects.

BHAGAVAD GITA 5:8–9

115.

Soul appears as a factor independent of the events in which we are immersed. Though I cannot identify soul with anything else, I also can never grasp it apart from other things, perhaps because it is like a reflection in a flowing mirror, or like the moon which mediates only borrowed light.

JAMES HILLMAN

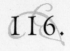

116.

WHO'S WATCHING?

Advanced yoga techniques can often serve to reinforce the ego. Who's watching? Whom do you hope to impress? If within the commitment to your yoga *sadhana* you drop the ego and the need for approval, you will create space for authenticity. Greeting your true Self as it is—you will become witness to all of your reality.

JR

117.

Contradictions have always existed in the soul of man. But it is only when we prefer analysis to silence that they become a constant and insoluble problem. We are not meant to resolve all contradictions but to live with them and rise above them.

WILLIAM BLAKE

118.

Here is a guide to finding a suitable teacher: he or she will have three simple but rare qualifications. One, they practice yoga themselves. Two, they have a good teacher themselves. Three, they care about you and are not arbitrarily imposing a standardized practice, philosophy or culture on you. Such a person can show you the yoga that is right for you. . . . The teacher is a friend. Someone you can trust, simply a friend, not the capital T teacher that spirituality would have us believe. This notion is fraught with the imbalance of power of someone knowing some "truth" that someone else does not know but is trying to get. This creates the imagined problem. . . .

With no roles being played it becomes apparent that student and teacher are obviously equal and share the same condition. In other words, "the guru's condition is my condition." Most spiritual teachers create a dynamic that prevents this, while paying lip service to the idea. Be cautious of anyone who cannot be this ordinary.

MARK WHITWELL

I19.

As soon as you trust yourself, you will know how to live.

GOETHE

I20.

The ritual process creates the safety, the predictable, the known. It may be the movements, chants or song that the group creates to start and end; it is a statement which acts as the container for change, for the journey, for the adventure.

SUE JENNINGS

121.

GAYATRI MANTRA

Om bhuh, bhuvaha swaha
Om Tat savitur varenyam
Bhargo devasya dhimahi
Dhiyo yonaha prachodayat

O self-effulgent light that has given birth to all the *lokas* (spheres of consciousness), who is worthy of worship and appears through the orbit of the sun, illumine our intellect.

RG. VEDA

122.

Practice *sadhana* as divine action. Engage in it for the sake of refining the action and not for its apparent results. Plant a seed for the joy of planting it. Living in *sadhana* brings alive your alliance with the cosmos. When you practice according to the cosmic rhythms and relinquish an expectation of control over your own life and nature, your sense of separation from the boundless presence of the Divine Mother evaporates, as do your personal grief and strife.

BRI MAYA TIWARI

123.

BREATH AND MOVEMENT

Breathe with attention to length of inhalation, length of exhalation, and retention of the breath while in moving sequences of postures or in stationary postures. Initiate the body movement with the breath movement. This *vinyasa* yields tremendous results.

JR

124.

Between this space is the *yoni* having its face towards the back; that space is called the root; there dwells the goddess Kundalini. It surrounds all the *nadis,* and has three coils and a half; and catching its tail in its mouth, it rests in the hole of *sushumna.*

It sleeps there like a serpent and is luminous by its own light. Like a serpent it lives between the joints; it is the goddess of speech and is called the seed (*bija*).

There, beautiful like the Bandhuk flower, is placed the seed of love; it is brilliant like burnished gold, and is described in Yoga as eternal.

The *sushumna* also embraced it, and the beautiful seed is there; there it rests shining brilliantly like the autumnal moon, with the luminosity of millions of suns, and the coolness of millions of moons. . . .

SIVA SAMHITA

125.

SITTING

Sitting after the physical practices allows me to absorb all the benefits of my good efforts. Now the mind is fit for concentration. Withdrawing the senses happens with ease. There is no need to strive. All is well. Meditation simply happens.

JR

126.

Our likes and dislikes, preferences and prejudices, like the concave and the convex lenses, distort the sameness of vision, the evenness of the mind which is so very essential to see things as they are, not as we want. The sameness of vision is Samadhi (merging the mind in Peace). Unless the mind is merged in the limitless Silence, in choiceless awareness, it is impossible to have the sameness of vision.

SWAMI NIRMALANANDA

127.

For the total development of the human being, solitude as a means of cultivating sensitivity becomes a necessity. One has to know what it means to be alone, what it is to meditate, what it is to die; and the implications of solitude, of meditation, of death, can be known only by seeking them out.

J. KRISHNAMURTI

128.

PURUSHA/PRAKRITI

Ancient concepts derived from the Samkhya school of philosophy, *purusha* and *prakriti*, have permeated yoga philosophy. In yoga, all of creation emanates from these two interdependent flows of existence. *Prakriti* means "excellent creation." Derived from *pra* (excellent) and *kriti* (creation). *Prakriti* represents undifferentiated phenomena (the world as we see it), outer nature, and that which is subject to change. Associated with the feminine, *prakriti* is the active creative force that makes life possible.

Purusha means the witness, the seer, the perceiver. That which does not change, that which is essential and supportive, is *purusha*. Likened to prana—invisible yet constant. Pure consciousness. Identifying with *purusha* reveals the Self in its essence. One stated aim of yoga practice is to reduce the clouds that veil a clear mind. When these subside we are given a glimpse of *purusha* and begin to perceive and operate from this place of pure, unobstructed consciousness. Identifying with *purusha* in no way diminishes *prakriti*; both are essential for maintaining the universe.

Practice

Sit in meditation. Notice that which is constant and that which changes. Experience your sense of both *purusha* (constancy) and *prakriti* (change).

JR

129.

Even after the Truth has been realized, there remains that strong, beginningless, obstinate impression that one is the agent and the experiencer, which is the cause of one's transmigration. It has to be carefully removed by living in a state of constant identification with the Supreme Self. Sages call that Liberation which is the attenuation of *vasanas* (impressions) here and now.

SRI SHANKARACHARYA

Overemphasis on individual development encouraged outside of the sacred circle has contributed significantly to the creation of unbearable rage, isolation and despair. In response, the desire to return to one's unquestioned place in the circle can be awakened. But we can easily romanticize possible membership in the collective without fully understanding the shadow aspects of belonging, why the circle has become absent. Our work in the Western world has been fiercely concerned with freeing the individual from the bonds of religious, political and familial rule. Accepting one's place in the circle could threaten this process of the development of the self. If membership is unconscious, the loss of freedom results. Unconscious commitment to a group ideology, participating in a mass psychology, means loss of freedom for all people involved.

Individualism, independence, even ego development, can threaten conscious membership in a collective when such processes are not in correct relationship to the whole. However, individuation, which is described by Jung as "coming into selfhood" or "self-realization" can enable us to richly and responsibly enter our place in the collective. Now our unprecedented task, perhaps unknown to our ancestors, is to bring the gifts of indi-

viduation into conscious membership in the whole, to find a way
to be uniquely ourselves inside a sacred, conscious circle.

JANET ADLER

131.

BHUVANESVARI

O Mother! Like the sleeping king of serpents,
Residing in the centre of the first lotus,
Thou didst create the universe
Thou dost ascend like a streak of lightning,
And attainist the ethereal region.

SIR JOHN WOODROFFE

132.

Yajnavalkya said: "I know that for many of you the real torment is that you must abandon your dear bodies. You imagine, not unreasonably, that the happiness of a disembodied spirit has something dreary about it. But that is not the case. After death, you will find yourself wandering through a haze, shouting without being heard, but all at once it will be you who hear. You will become aware that someone is following you, like an animal in the forest, only now in the darkness of the heavens. The person following you is your oblation, the being composed of the offering you made in your life. In a whisper, he will say to you: "Come here, come here, it is I, your Self." And in the end you will follow him.

ROBERTO CALASSO

133.

VRIKSASANA—TREE POSE

The tree is our great teacher. An ancient symbol of regeneration in many cultures, the tree links the underworld, the earth, and the heavens. The roots coming up through the earth represent the unconscious or hidden aspects of the self that emerge into light as the trunk and branches on the visible plane.

The tree is associated with the Great Goddess. Early depictions of Mother Mary show her flowing form coming out of a tree. Cross-culturally, the tree has been seen as a metaphor for the human body. When we embody the tree in yoga, we re-create the ancient mystical practices of nature worship and develop reverence for the world around us. Sage Bhagiratha performed the tree balance as a way to influence the descent of the Ganges to earth during drought.

In the tree pose we feel the ground beneath the feet, strength in the trunk, and the yielding nature of the leaves and branches. The seasonal fluctuations of old leaves falling and new leaves growing inspire us to accept life's changes and to let go of the past. In practicing the tree pose, we honor the interrelatedness of human and plant life. We also continue the lineage of tree worship, thus directly acknowledging our reliance on trees for life itself.

JR

134.

The first indication of the coming of Spiritual Consciousness is the dawning perception of the reality of the Ego—the awareness of the real existence for the Soul. When one begins to feel that he *himself* is his soul, rather than that he possesses a wonderful something called the "soul" of which he really knows nothing—when we say, he feels that he *is* a soul, rather than that he *has* or *will have* a soul—then that one is nearing the first stages of Spiritual Consciousness if indeed he is not already within its outer borders.

YOGI RAMACHARAKA

135.

The greatness of a nation and its moral progress can be judged by the way its animals are treated.

GANDHI

136.

SAGE PATANJALI

Srimatye, Anantaya, Nagarajaya, Namo Namaha

INVOCATION TO PATANJALI

The author of *The Yoga Sutras*, Patanjali is known as an incarnation of Ananta—the "Endless One," the serpent god of eternity. A cobra's hood hangs like a canopy above his head, reminiscent of the *naga* tribes of southern India.

The *nagas* were known as divine serpent people and worshiped as protectors of rivers, streams, and wells. *Nagas* could bring rain and promote fertility, or, in their destructive aspect, unleash floods and drought. Their dual creative and destructive roles link them to Devi, the Great Goddess, who must be appeased with ritual offerings, lest she destroy that which she creates. *Nagas* also symbolize Narayana (Vishnu), who sleeps upon the coiled body of Adisesha who is king of the Cobras, thus linking Patanjali to the worship of Vishnu.

Practice

The practice of bhujangasana (the cobra pose) links us to the great *naga* beings, to Vishnu, to the Mother Goddess, and to Patanjali himself.

JR

137.

Is obedience to the teacher a way of dealing with ego and personal desire?

Yes. The tradition prescribes that. To ward away the ego you have to have obedience to the teacher. And this teacher is none other than your own Self.

You have to be obedient to that which you are seeking.

However, A TRUE TEACHER DOES NOT EXPECT OBEDIENCE FROM ANYBODY.

ELI-JAXON BEAR

SATSANG WITH H. W. L. POONJA

138.

God, or enlightenment, is the ultimate pleasure, uninterrupted happiness. No such thing exists. Your wanting something that does not exist is the root of your problem. Transformation, *moksha*, liberation, and all that stuff are just variations of the same theme: permanent happiness. The body can't take uninterrupted pleasure for long; it would be destroyed. Wanting to impose a fictitious permanent state of happiness on the body is a serious neurological problem.

U. G. KRISHNAMURTI

139.

If you have come to help me, you are wasting your time. But if you have come because your liberation is bound up with mine, then let us work together.

AUSTRALIAN ABORIGINAL WOMAN

140.

PRACTICE TIME

Q: Dr. Kabat-Zinn, how long should I practice for?
A: How should I know?

JON KABAT-ZINN

Kabat-Zinn's response flips the question back to the student. Yoga students tend to turn this question around, asking the teacher: "How long do *you* practice each day?" The student is often tempted to measure herself by an outside standard rather than going inward and finding out what is needed day to day. Yoga in its pure form is outside of temporal reality. What is a minute or an hour to one totally absorbed in a state of yoga?

A few minutes of genuine body/breath/mind integration is more worthwhile than one or two hours of advanced asana performed without regard to the breath and with a scattered mind.

Try to see yoga practice as quality of attention rather than quantity of minutes, and you might just find that you have lost track of time altogether.

JR

141.

To take responsibility for facing our living condition, we must look at who we are and how we see the world. Every day, we wake up in the morning and are hit by the biggest intuitive lie known to human consciousness. That lie goes like this: "It's me, it's me, I'm it, I'm the center of the universe. I come first. I hold it all together." The bottom line is "me." It is not just that we are selfish; it is deeper. We perceive the self as the one sure thing, the only thing, that we can count on. I am sure of my own ideas, my own dictates. I know without question what I want, what I hate, what I fear. I think, therefore I am. . . . Such self-involvement is natural, given that we see ourselves as the most important thing in the universe. Moral condemnation of it is beside the point. But I question its accuracy. While we may wake up "knowing" that we're the center of the universe, the minute we walk outside we will not encounter one single person who agrees with us.

ROBERT THURMAN

142.

Mind is interested in what happens,
while awareness is interested in the mind itself.
The child is after the toy, but the mother watches the
child, not the toy.

SRI NISARGADATTA MAHARAJ

143.

LET IT BE NOW

A yoga friend really wanted to push herself in her practice. She described an "adjustment" (physical manipulation in a pose) made by her teacher. Through this manipulation, she could hear and feel an opening in her heart chakra—a literal popping open of her sternum that brought her deeper into back bends and deeper into bliss. She yearned for more of this blissful intensity and seemed disappointed when it didn't recur. In chasing after an experience and trying to repeat a sensation, she was living in the past. (You may find that you do this in yoga or in other aspects of your life.) Her body rebelled and did not deliver this sought-after experience. She became disappointed. In seeking, she interfered with the process of yoga, which only exists in the present, NOW.

Practice

Have you ever tried to replicate the sensation of a pose from one day to the next? Our bodies are living, breathing animals subject to change. When your teacher helps you into a pose, do you feel frustrated that you can't "get" that feeling on your own? The more we chase after an experience, the more it eludes us. Remember John Lennon and Paul McCartney's words of wisdom, and let it be, NOW.

JR

144.

There is a strange tree, which stands without roots and
  bears
fruits without blossoming;
It has no branches and no leaves, it is lotus all over.
Two birds sing there; one is the Guru, and the other the
  disciple:
The disciple chooses the manifold fruits of life and
  tastes them,
and the Guru beholds him in joy.
What Kabir says is hard to understand: "The bird is
  beyond seeking, yet it is most clearly visible. The
  Formless is in the midst of all forms. I sing the glory
  of forms."

KABIR

145.

Fortunately (psycho) analysis is not the only way to resolve inner conflicts. Life itself still remains a a very effective therapist.

KAREN HORNEY

146.

The *knowledge* of *knowledge compels*. It compels us to adopt an attitude of permanent vigilance against the temptation of certainty. It compels us to recognize that certainty is not a proof of truth. It compels us to realize that the world everyone sees is not *the* world but *a* world . . . If we know that our world is necessarily the world we bring forth with others, every time we are in conflict with another human being *with whom we want to remain in coexistence,* we cannot affirm what for us is certain (an absolute truth) because that would negate the other person. If we want to coexist with the other person, we must see that *his certainty—however undesirable it may seem to us—is as legitimate and valid as our own.* . . . Hence the only possibility for coexistence is to opt for a broader perspective, a domain of existence—in which both parties fit in the bringing forth of a common world.

FRANCISCO VARELA AND HUMBERTO MATURANA

147.

As we favour hands and brain hemispheres, so we favour other organs. Each of us favours particular glands; hormones and even thoughts and images; we *favour* them, preferring them to other tissues and concepts in the organization of our lives. Modern medicine considers variations in susceptibility to certain illnesses—for example, proposing that so-called Type A people are more likely than the general population to suffer form peptic ulcers and hypertension—but Ayurveda has synthesized metabolic tendencies and character traits into a system. It is not a clean, quantifiable system that can plot your existence with clinical precision, because such straight line graphs cannot accurately represent human systems; humans are better represented as complex waves generated by the force of ego's gravity trying to keep the individual functioning as a well-integrated unit.

ROBERT SVOBODA

148.

Darkness cannot drive out darkness; only light can do that.

Hate cannot drive out hate; only love can do that. Hate multiplies hate, violence multiplies violence, and toughness multiplies toughness in a descending spiral of destruction . . .

The chain reaction of evil—hate begetting hate,

wars producing more wars—must be broken, or we shall be plunged into the darkness of annihilation.

DR. MARTIN LUTHER KING, JR.

149.

TIME'S NECTAR

Amrita, the life-giving nectar, is housed in the third eye center. As we age, it descends drop by drop into the fire of the solar plexus and burns up there. When we turn upside down in inverted poses, the flow of this sacred nectar reverses itself and remains stored in the third eye known as the *anja chakra.* This protects the body from the progress of time and bestows bliss. This in part may explain why inverted poses like the shoulder stand feel so powerful.

JR

150.

Talk Talk
No matter what the subject of the conversation
the illuminated person talks only of GOD.

No matter what the subject matter,
even if the conversation is about GOD,
the ordinary man talks only about himself.

JONATHAN LEWIS

151.

YOGA SUTRAS

The sage Patanjali distilled the teachings of yoga into a concise text
of aphorisms known as *The Yoga Sutras*. Sutra means thread. In this
text, Patanjali weaves each thread together to create the essence

of yoga. He divides this text into four chapters: Concentration, Means/Practice, Extraordinary Powers, and Absolute Freedom. Patanjali brings the various ancient teachings of yoga to their core purpose, creating a tangible road to spiritual freedom through his precise and sparse language. The *Sutras* were designed to create a dialogue between student and teacher and to deepen that relationship. For anyone willing to look into the nature of his or her own mind, *The Yoga Sutras* provide the means. They also provide hope for the soul's liberation.

JR

152.

The posture of yoga is steady and easy.
It is realized by relaxing one's effort and resting like
the cosmic serpent on the waters of infinity.
Then one is unconstrained by opposing dualities.

YOGA SUTRA OF PATANJALI II:46–48

153.

When you truly feel equal love for all beings, when your heart has expanded so much that it embraces the whole of creation, you will certainly not feel like giving up this or that. You will simply drop off from secular life as a ripe fruit drops from the branch of a tree. You will feel that the whole world is your home.

SRI RAMANA MAHARSHI

154.

Commentary and translation stand in the same relation to the text as style and mimesis to nature: the same phenomenon considered from different aspects. On the tree of the sacred text both are the eternally rustling leaves; on that of the profane, the seasonally falling fruits.

WALTER BENJAMIN

155.

The Body is the sacred field of Kashi.

All pervading wisdom is the Ganges, Mother of the
   Three Worlds.

Devotion and faith—these are Gaya.

Devout meditation on the feet of one's own *guru*—

This is Prayaga.

And the highest state of consciousness, the inner-soul,
   this witness of the hearts of all people—
      this is Vishvesha, the Lord of All.

If all this dwells within my body,

What other place of pilgrimage can there be?

SRI SHANKARACHARYA

156.

Before we know to question, to agree or disagree, we must first understand what the teacher is offering. In Yoga, this further means to engage practices we are taught, whether physical, mental, or spiritual. Only through accepting the *experience* of the teaching can we know if it is of value to us. It was only because my father (T. Krishnamacharya) accepted and fully comprehended the lessons of his teachers that the he was able to adapt and change their knowledge for the present and future.

T. K. V. DESIKACHAR

157.

Disappointment is the best chariot to use on the path of the *dharma*. It does not confirm the existence of our ego and its dreams. However, if we are involved with spiritual materialism, if we regard spirituality as a part of our accumulation of learning and virtue, if spirituality becomes a way of building ourselves up, then of course the whole process of surrendering is completely distorted. If we regard spirituality as a way of making ourselves comfortable, then whenever we experience something unpleasant, a disappointment, we try to rationalize it . . . We dare not contemplate any other way. We develop the conviction that whatever we experience is part of our spiritual development. "I've made it, I have experienced it, I am a self-made person and I know everything, roughly, because I've read books and they confirm *my* beliefs, my rightness, my ideas. Everything coincides."

CHOGYAM TRUNGPA

158.

EIGHT LIMBS

Patanjali presents the eight limbs of yoga known as ashtanga in *The Yoga Sutras.* This system gives the practitioner the tools to achieve profound peace, which comes from merging with the object of contemplation. The first four limbs of yoga can be practiced. These are: yama, niyama, asana, and pranayama. These preparatory stages make it more likely that the last four stages of pratyahara , dharana, dhyana, and samadhi will unfold. These last four result from steady practice or can even occur spontaneously.

While the eight limbs of Patanjali's Yoga have an intentional design, the progression through them need not be linear. The principles of ashtanga center on Self-knowledge and devotion to ishvara, the spiritual principle (God). The connection between daily life, our relationships with self and others, and our yoga practice deepens as the journey into ashtanga unfolds. While tremendously popular in the West, yoga postures (asanas) are but one eighth of Patanjali's Yoga.

OUTLINE OF THE EIGHT LIMBS

Yama

This first limb of Yoga concerns our relationships with others and with the world at large. Yamas describe ethical and moral guidelines for self-conduct and are subdivided into:

ahimsa: nonviolence
satya: truthfulness
asteya: nonstealing

brahmacharya: continence
aparigraha: noncovetousness

Niyama

This second limb concerns the relationship we have with ourselves.

The five niyamas are:

saucha: cleanliness
samtosha: contentment
tapas: heat; spiritual austerities
svadhyaya: self-study (through observation and study)
isvara pranidhana: surrender to God

Asana

This third limb means seat or body posture.

Pranayama

The fourth limb means literally "life force extension" and refers to special breathing practices.

Pratyahara

The fifth limb means withdrawal of the senses from the outer world and moving them inward.

Dharana
Concentration is the sixth limb.

Dhyana
Meditation is the seventh limb.

Samadhi
This final limb is known as contemplation, integration, or perfection of concentration.

JR

159.

The great error of this age is that activity has increased so much that there is little margin left in one's everyday life for repose. Repose is the secret of all contemplation and meditation, the secret of getting in tune with that aspect of life which is the essence of all things. When one is not accustomed to take repose, one does not know what is behind one's being.

HAZRAT INAYAT KHAN

160.

He who thinks he knows It not, knows It. He who thinks he knows It, knows It not. The true knowers think they can never know It (because of Its infinitude), while the ignorant think they know It.

KENA UPANISHAD

161.

WHO MOVES? WHO BREATHES?

Today there is no practice. No doing of practice.
No moving, no breathing, and no doing of moving/
    breathing.
Now
I feel moved.
I am
moved.

No distinctions or duality
just breath moving me. No struggle. No me.
Only this one gift of breath
Moving me.

JR

162.

TRIPUTA

Such as recite thy primordial golden *bija*
SRIM
Attain all prosperity and fortune

O Mother!
He who contemplates Thy second *bija*
Adorned by numbers of Devas,
HRIM
gains all prosperity.

The chiefs of men who meditate upon Thy *bija*,
Lustrous as the sun,
KLIM
Charm the three worlds
And by recitation thereof become like unto Isvawara.

SIR JOHN WOODROFFE

163.

When we use mantra, it is better to master the vibratory effect in
the whole body before meaning is attributed. The single point of
focus is the sound itself. Om means Om and Ma is Ma; we are
linked directly without the filtering mechanism of mind.

MARK WHITWELL

164.

There are no good pupils, there are only good teachers. Teaching is not an imposition of the teacher's will over that of the pupil, not at all. Teaching starts with freedom and ends with freedom.

VANDA SCARAVELLI

165.

Mind's whole function is to go on dividing. The function of the heart is to see the joining link about which the mind is completely blind.

OSHO

166.

The kind of heightened sensitivity that results from yoga practice means more awareness of pain as well as pleasure. When the ego reacts to this possibility from the standpoint of fear, we will tend to opt for less rather than more feeling, and, expecting the worst, begin to harden ourselves. We then build *up* our ego defenses, some of which can actually mask as ego-inflation. Several religious techniques of prayer and meditation that deny body and the feelings have developed within various traditions, all in the name of detachment or some similar notion of transcendence. Even yoga can be misused in this way. Because it involves development of the will, yoga can easily degenerate into an exercise to prove that the will can suppress all feeling in order to obtain a kind of superhuman status. But attempting to attain the status of a god without understanding what it means to be human is a travesty of the Spirit. Denial of emotion in the name of God or any other power only prolongs ignorance and suffering of the self and others.

ROXANNE KAMAYANI GUPTA

167.

We must learn in our performance of asanas to express the outer form and beauty of the pose without losing our inner attention. The skin is an organ of perception. It does not act. It receives. All actions are received by the skin, but if your flesh overstretches when you are performing an asana, the skin loses its sensitivity and sends no message to the brain. In the West, you tend to overdo the stretch. You want to get something. You want to do it quickly. You want to succeed in doing the pose, but you don't feel the reaction. The flesh extends so much that it makes the organ of perception insensitive, and because it has become insensitive, the reflection from the action to the mind is not felt.

B. K. S. IYENGAR

168.

NAD YOGA

Indian philosophy teaches that all material existence is preceded by and composed of sound vibration. The world literally comes from sound. Sanskrit mantras are repeated words or phrases that form a link with the divine and invoke the wisdom of the ancients. Chanting mantras open all chakras and cleanse the mind. Many mantras can be traced back thousands of years to the Rg. Veda, India's oldest known sacred text. The OM mantra, which re-creates the sound of the universe, is imbued with meaning and is simultaneously without meaning. OM invokes the pulse of pure being and gives shape to breath. Yoga too is deeply steeped in elements of sound, mostly through mantras and recitation of sacred texts.

-Work with a mantra that is specific to your needs.
-Consult with your teacher to find a mantra that is appropriate for you.

JR

169.

Many people believe that the practice of yoga is concerned with "making your mind a blank"—a condition which could, if it were really desirable, be much more easily achieved by asking a friend to hit you over the head with a hammer . . . (However, what we are really trying to do is) to unlearn the false identification of the thought-waves with the ego-sense.

CHRISTOPHER ISHERWOOD AND
SWAMI PRABHAVANANDA

170.

This Self is never born, nor does It die. It did not spring from anything, nor did anything spring from It. This Ancient One is unborn, eternal, everlasting. It is not slain even though the body is slain.

KATHA UPANISHAD

171.

MOUSE WHISKER
OR PINHOLE

The space between my thoughts is as narrow as a mouse whisker and as tiny as a pinhole. Or there is no space at all—mind hijacked by overlapping monkey banter, whooping in my ear. In yoga, that same space opens as wide as the ocean and as silent as the deepest sea.

JR

172.

If I speak in the tongues of men and of angels, but have not love, I am only a resounding gong or a clanging cymbal. If I have the gift of prophecy and can fathom all mysteries and all knowledge, and if I have a faith that can move mountains, but have not love, I am nothing. . . .

Now we see but a poor reflection as in a mirror; then we shall see face to face. Now I know in part. Then I shall know fully, even as I am fully known.

And now these three remain: faith, hope and love. But the greatest of these is love.

I CORINTHIANS

173.

(This) variety of meanings corresponds to a real morphological diversity. If the word "yoga" means many things, that is because yoga is many things.

MIRCEA ELIADE

174.

The training process in (such) Asian disciplines is not simply like ritual process, it is ritual process. The result may be just as radical and effective transformation of the individual as what occurs in healing or life-cycle rituals.

P. ZARRILI

175.

The other kind of concentration is that in which the consciousness contains no object—only subconscious impressions, which are like burnt seeds. It is attained by constantly checking the thought waves through the practice of non-attachment.

YOGA SUTRA I:18

176.

SAMSKARA

The Sanskrit term *samskara* translates as activator. *Samskara* is like a groove on a record turning around and around in which the needle gets stuck or like an old tape that plays in our mind turning over the same thoughts, impressions, and memories. *Samskara* is a cycle of action and thought that becomes our habits. These habits often feel like fated repetitions. When we feel stuck, it is

often due to *samskara*. Obsessions and compulsions have their
root in the *samskara* of past conditioning, but they can also produce positive tendencies like our life's work, the ability to sustain
relationships, and the soul's longing for the divine.

Yoga, in the broadest sense of both practice and theory, concerns itself with the molding of *samskara*. Refining *samskara* to such
a degree that it becomes a positive force that guides life and energy
is yoga. This requires self-inquiry. If approached with this kind of
awareness, the practice of asana takes on new meaning and new life.

JR

177.

Your children are not your children.
They are the sons and daughters of Life's longing for
 itself.
They come through you but not from you,
And though they are with you yet they belong not to
 you.

You may give them your love but not your thoughts,
For they have their own thoughts.
You may house their bodies but not their souls,
For their souls dwell in the house of tomorrow, which
    you cannot visit, not even
in your dreams.
You may strive to be like them, but seek
not to make them like you.
For life goes not backward nor tarries
with yesterday.

KHALIL GIBRAN

178.

The Hatha Yoga can not be obtained without the Raja Yoga, nor
can the Raja Yoga be obtained without the Hatha Yoga. Therefore
let the Yogi first learn the Hatha Yoga from the instructions of
the wise Guru.

SIVA SAMHITA

179.

GRATITUDE

My inner smile widens. I am greeted by a roomful of people who choose to come together in yoga. To celebrate the body together in a feast of souls called "yoga class" gives shape and meaning to my days. An electrical charge runs through me brightly; Kundalini at work generates new and old approaches to poses, to breath, to life.

Together we salute the sun daily, the moon too. We re-create the world of nature; the elements, animals, fish, moon and stars, plants and herbs, geometrical shapes, and poses of great sages and children. Gratitude for this day of work, of play. Gratitude.

JR

180.

THE TRADITION

No one behind, no one ahead.
The path the ancients cleared has closed. And the other
    path, everyone's path, easy and
wide, goes nowhere.
I am alone and find my way.

DHARMAKIRTI

181.

That's why in the Hindu system, a mystic word, or *mantram*, is given to the student to repeat. The meaning of *mantram* is "that which keeps the mind steady and produces the proper effect." Its repetition is called *japa* . . . It is not somehere outside but always within. Wherever you are, your *mantram* is with you.

SRI SWAMI SATCHIDANANDA

182.

Persevering practice will support you more than a thousand hours of armchair philosophy.

JR

183.

SURYA NAMASKAR—SALUTATION TO THE SUN

Practiced in conjunction with the rising sun, surya namaskar links asanas in a steady flow honoring the gifts of the sun god, Surya. Traditionally, invocations in the form of chants to the sun were uttered while practicing the body movements.

Surya namaskar begins with the hands assuming the gesture of prayer and continues through an endless variety of full body asanas in a steady flow linking body and breath. Here we give thanks for the gifts of life bestowed upon us by the sun and all the planets. Surya namaskar is the foundation of many yoga practices. When performed with a sense of *bhava* (feeling, devotion) it raises the level of practice from the mere physical and temporal to that of the eternal.

JR

184.

Homage to the Breath of Life, for this whole universe
   obeys it,
Which has become the Lord of all, on which all things
   are based.
O Breath of Life, that form of thine so dear,
O Breath of Life, that form which is yet dearer,
And then that healing which (too) is thine
Place it in us that we may live.

ATHARVA-VEDA

185.

Sow love, reap peace . . .
Sow meditation, reap wisdom.

SWAMI SIVANANDA

186.

Being able to process the raw, chaotic vibrations of the "quantum soup" and turn them into meaningful, orderly bits of reality opens up enormous creative possibilities. However, these possibilities exist only when you are aware of them. . . . (These) automatic processes play a huge part in aging, for as we age, our ability to coordinate these functions declines. A lifetime of unconscious living leads to numerous deteriorations, while a lifetime of conscious participation prevents them. The very act of paying conscious attention to bodily functions instead of leaving them on automatic pilot will change how you age. Every so-called involuntary function, from heartbeat and breathing to digestion and hormone regulation, can be consciously controlled.

DEEPAK CHOPRA

187.

The nature of spiritual devotion is the supreme love.
And its essence is the nectar of immortality.
Because there is no difference between the grace of God
and those great souls arising from that grace
Cultivate grace alone; cultivate grace alone.

BHAKTI NARADA SUTRAS

188.

KURMASANA—TORTOISE

According to the Hindu Vedas, the tortoise known as Kurma (the second incarnation of Vishnu) supports the entire world upon his back. After the great deluge in which many of the sacred Vedic teachings were destroyed, Kurma swam to the bottom of the sea, carrying the huge Mount Meru. A snake was tied around the mountain and together they were used by the gods to churn the ocean in search of the lost *amrita* (nectar of immortality). Through their joint efforts the nectar of the lost teachings was recovered and the Gods retained their immortality.

Practice
The pose of the tortoise, known as Kurmasana, requires that while folding forward, the ankles wrap around the head and the hands interlace behind the back. As we draw into ourselves like a tortoise into its shell, we cultivate introspection and the ability to hold things together.

JR

189.

There are no accidents only incidents.
Life is a series of incidents.

SWAMI DAYANANDA SARASWATI

190.

I cannot imagine anything more noble or more national than that for, say, one hour in the day, we should all do the labour that the poor must do, and thus identify ourselves with them and through them with all mankind. I cannot imagine a better workshop of God than that in His name I should labour for the poor even as they do.

GANDHI

191.

A fourth type of breath control goes beyond the range of exhalation and inhalation. Then the cover over the light of truth dissolves. And the mind is fit for concentration.

YOGA SUTRA OF PATANJALI II:51–53

192.

LIFESAVING PRESENCE

As a seasoned yoga teacher, I have heard many people proclaim, "Yoga saved my life!" The stories and people are unique, yet the conviction is always the same: "I couldn't have survived without yoga."

When I hear how yoga helps overcome the pain of injuries, accidents, illness, and emotional upheaval, I stand in awe. No longer an "it," yoga stops feeling like a mere routine, an entertaining form of exercise, or another spiritual "pursuit." It has become a living presence among us—touching and often healing those who come in contact with its power. When someone declares, "Yoga saved my life," what she means is "I saved my own life." She has reassembled what has fallen apart. The miraculous power of yoga does not sit out there in some ancient system of philosophy and body exercises. It's directly here and now inside the heart. Inside your core, your own true Self.

JR

193.

My inward petition was instantly acknowledged. First a delightful cool wave descended under my back and over my feet, banishing all discomfort. Then, to my amazement, the temple became greatly magnified. Its large door opened slowly, revealing the stone figure of the goddess Kali. Gradually the statue changed into a living form, smiling, nodding in greeting, thrilling me with joy indescribable. As if by a mystic syringe, the breath was withdrawn from my lungs; my body became very still, though not inert. An ecstatic enlargement of consciousness followed. I could see clearly for several miles over the Ganges River to my left, and beyond the temple into the entire Dakshineswar precinct. The walls of all the buildings glimmered transparently; through them I observed people walking to and fro over distant acres.

PARAMAHAMSA YOGANANDA

194.

It is only with the heart that one can see rightly; what is essential is invisible to the eye.

ANTOINE DE SAINT-EXUPÉRY

195.

ARDHA CHANDRASANA—THE HALF-MOON POSE

The copper-colored moon god, Chandra (also known as Soma), makes the evening dew that falls upon the plants. According to legend, when taken as a drink this Soma becomes a powerful ambrosia for men, women, and gods by inducing awesome strength, hallucinations, and immortality. As we practice the half-moon pose, ardha chandrasana, we can imagine the gravitational pull of the moon and dive into the powerful forces that moon energy symbolizes. We cultivate balance and strength as we land in the pose perched on one leg and arm.

Practice
    -For calming and cooling and to ease anxiety visualize
     the moon.
    -Practice the half-moon pose on full and new lunar days.
    -Create a full-moon and new-moon meditation.

JR

196.

I come into the earth and with life giving love I support all things on earth. And I become the scent and taste of the sacred plant Soma, which is the wandering moon.

BHAGAVAD GITA 15:13

197.

Alchemy and medicine originated as necessary aids to the fulfillment of spiritual objectives.

Hindu alchemy can be traced back to the Vedic period. The Rig
Veda describes the Soma Rasa, or the juice of the Soma plant, as
amrita, which is akin to the Greek ambrosia. In spite of the diver-
gence of views as to the attributes and properties of Soma, it is
generally agreed that it must have been an extremely potent eu-
phoriant. Authorities agree that it was a milky climbing plant,
most probably Asclepias Acida or Ephedra or a type of unculti-
vated vine. For the extraction of juice, Soma herbs were crushed
between two stones or pounded in a mortar; the extracted liquid
was then filtered through sheep's wool and subsequently mixed
with milk, butter or honey. The texts describe its reaction on the
body as no less than a "roar of a bull." Soma was an inexhaustible
source of strength and vitality: it increased sexual energy, stimulated speech and possessed healing properties.

AJIT MOOKERJEE AND MADHU KHANNA

198.

Know thou the self (*atman*) as riding in a chariot,
The body as the chariot.
Know thou the intellect (*buddhi*) as the chariot-driver,
And the mind as the reins.
The senses, they say, are the horses;
The objects of sense, what they range over.
The self combined with senses and mind
Wise men call "the enjoyer."
He however who has not understanding,
Who is unmindful and ever impure,
Reaches not the goal,
But goes on to transmigration (rebirth).
He, however, who has understanding,
Who is mindful and ever pure,
Reaches the goal
From which he is born no more.

KATHA UPANISHAD

199.

GEOGRAPHY OF THE BODY

The sacred geography of the body is viewed by yoga texts and Vedanta as a microcosm of the universe. The body itself becomes a temple, and thus the need for external places of worship becomes superfluous. Ancient practitioners used forests and caves as places of meditation, relying on the inner sanctum to meet God—their own true Self.

JR

200.

How wonderful that we have met with a paradox. Now we have some hope of making progress.

NIELS BOHR

201.

THE GREAT RELIGIONS

The
Great religions are the
Ships,
Poets the life
Boats.
Every sane person I know has jumped
Overboard.
That is good for business
Isn't it
Hafiz?

HAFIZ

202.

Under these circumstances, the life that we live is a contradiction and a conflict. Because consciousness *must* involve both pleasure and pain, to strive for pleasure to the exclusion of pain is, in effect, to strive for the loss of consciousness. Because such a loss is in principle the same as death, this means that the more we struggle for life (as pleasure), the more we are actually killing what we love.

ALAN WATTS

203.

We take our first, faltering gasp of air the moment we leave the womb. We draw life into us in the early years of childhood, youth, and early adulthood as we learn, discover our nature, find our place in the world: our *dharma*. In its fulfillment, we begin to give back all that we are capable of, all that we can offer to others. As a long expiration, we gradually give back the breath of life and consciousness, returning it to the source, to God.

T. K. V. DESIKACHAR

204.

SITTING BUDDHA

Buddha sits under the *boddhi* tree in deep yogic trance. Having attained enlightenment, he serves as a model for all yoga practitioners. Sitting meditation encourages inner stillness, and Buddha reminds us of our potential for silence and freedom on all levels. A Buddhalike mind, trained inward, results from practice or may arise spontaneously. The focused mind opens the way for meditation, awareness, and right action. Through our practice, the heart blossoms like a lotus and our capacity for love and compassion becomes limitless.

JR

205.

In the West everyone has to *learn* everything. There has to be a manual. Do this, then do that, then stand on your head, then breath in and out . . . My dear sir, just look at Ma. Doesn't some sort of love spring up in your heart? Well then, follow that love, however small it is. It will take you to a fountain. All you have to do then is sit in the fountain and get cool.

MR. REDDY IN *HIDDEN JOURNEY*, BY ANDREW HARVEY

206.

I would a hundred times rather have a little heart and no brain, than be all brains and no heart . . . He who has no heart and only brain dies of dryness.

SWAMI VIVEKANANDA

207.

OM

Repetition of the sound OM reveals its meaning.

YOGA SUTRA OF PATANJALI

In *The Yoga Sutras*, OM is known as *pranava*. In chanting OM, the sound is really more like AUM. With the first "Ah" we activate the entire chakra system and set in motion AUM's journey through all seven chakras. The next sound of "ooo" fills the body between the root and crown chakras and finally "mmm" completes the journey by flowing out into the infinite. This journey repeats itself time and again.

Listen for the primordial sound of the universe pulsating in the sound OM. Through OM ishvara manifests in sound and connects us to something that transcends the questioning duality of mind. By chanting OM we bring the sacred into our heart. Persevere with this mantra and the result will be peace and tranquillity. Layers of meaning will be revealed through the sound vibrating in the body, which opens up to the mystery of all life.

Practice
- Find your way into the meaning of the sound OM by constant repetition.
- Frame your yoga practice with three or more OMs chanted at the start and finish of asana, pranayama, and meditation practice.
- Use OM to focus your mind during asana or meditation.
- Count OMs as you inhale or exhale.

JR

208.

Yoga is Self-love.

SWAMI DAYANANDA SARASWATI

209.

A thoughtless man having identified with his thoughts, is carried away by his mind like a drifting piece of wood and he is tosssed hither and thither by its various urges, whereas a thoughtful person carefully watches the movement of his mind without identifying himself, with any of his thoughts. Such alert but passive observation without identification with thoughts brings about an inner awakening which becomes the guiding light of peace and understanding.

SWAMI NIRMALANANDA

210.

Stop seeking. Where is there to go? Everything you seek is already inside of you.

JR

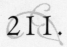

211.

Yogis should meditate like this: in your navel is a lotus surmounted by a sun disc, whereupon is an inverted triangle which is formed of the three *gunas*. In the middle is the great goddess Chinnamasta blazing as a flame, unequalled and incomparable. She is established in the *yoni* mudra and her eyes are directed to her heart.

CHINNAMASTATANTRA

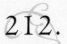

212.

Two birds, fast bound companions,
Clasp close the self-same tree.
Of those two, the one eats sweet fruit;
the other looks on without eating.

MUNDUKYA UPANISHAD

213.

There exists today a kind of Yoga Fundamentalism, which has two wings, that we will call Literalism and Relativism. They masquerade in many forms with many doctrines and techniques. They stain the work of both traditional and concocted methods of practice and they produce more in the way of politics, self-righteousness and avoidance than they do happiness. There also exists a resolution to this Fundamentalism's Two Wings. However, it is not a system, a doctrine or a technique. It is more practically a magic ingredient that refines a system or technique, so that we are able to perform its methods skillfully (even artistically) and then step out of them, free and unbiased.

RICHARD FREEMAN

214.

There was a cowherd boy who took his cows to the meadows every morning and brought them back to the cowshed at the end of the day. One evening, as he was tying the cows up for the night, the boy found that one of them was missing her rope. He feared that she might run away, but it was too late to go and buy a new rope. The boy didn't know what to do, so he went to a wise man who lived nearby and sought his advice. The wise man told the boy to pretend to tie the cow, and make sure that the cow saw him doing it. The boy did as the wise man suggested and pretended to tie the cow. The next morning the boy discovered that the cow had remained still throughout the night. He untied all the cows as usual, and they all went outside. He was about to go to the meadows when he noticed that the cow with the missing rope was still in the cowshed. She was standing on the same spot where she had been all night. He tried to coax her to join the herd, but she wouldn't budge. The boy was perplexed. He went back to the wise man who said,

"The cow still thinks she is tied up. Go back and pretend to untie her."

The boy did as he was told, and the cow happily left the cowshed. This is what the guru does with the ego of the disciple. The guru helps untie that which was never there. Like the cow, due to our ignorance, we believe that we are bound by the ego when, in fact, we are completely free. We need to be convinced of this, however.

SRI MATA AMRITANANDAMAYI (AMMACHI)

215.

WHEN THINGS FALL APART

Things fall apart. The center cannot hold.

WILLIAM BUTLER YEATS

When things fall apart yoga can help. Yoga works from the inside helping us confront things we might prefer to ignore. Like a mirror, the practice throws back a clear reflection and yoga can also act as a balm. So, in times of crisis, take refuge in yoga. Let it soothe you as it heals you. Things do fall apart every day. But they come together again with the inner movement called yoga.

JR

216.

Indian music—the very blessing of the Divine as Siva—has given us the gift of the *tambura*, the four stringed *veena* or drone, which gives you a feeling of groundedness, so you do not get lost as in Western music. The *tambura* will support you always. It is said that even Saraswati, goddess of wisdom and learning and music, when she enters the Nada Brahman, the ocean of sound, feels that it is so impenetrable, so profound, that she is concerned lest she, the goddess of music, may be lost, inundated by it. So she places two gourds around her, in the form of *veena*, and then she is guided by them into it (the ocean of sound).

SRI KARUNAMAYEE

217.

Do your practice and all is coming.

K. PATTABHI JOIS

218.

Ganesha is sometimes mistakenly thought of as the "remover" of obstacles. While it is true that he is most often supplicated to remove obstacles, it is more accurate to recognize him as Vighnesha, the "Lord of Obstacles." He may remove them, or he may pose them. He may open the door or close it. Ganesha may be chubby, good-humored, always carrying a radish in one hand and a plate of sweetmeats in the other. But he may also be the stern doorkeeper of the universe, with his elephant goad, his noose and his hatchet. As Lord of Obstacles, Ganesha sits at the threshold, especially at the threshold of the sacred.

DIANA ECK

219.

Traditionally it is said that for a real practitioner, it's not the negative experiences but the good ones that bring obstacles. When things are going well you have to be especially careful and mindful so that you don't become complacent or over-confident . . . What we have to learn in both meditation and in life, is to be free of attachment to the good experiences and free of aversion to the negative ones.

SOGYAL RINPOCHE

220.

SAMTOSHA

How quickly do you want to flip to the next page? To run from one thing to another? Like a fly, are you always seeking, always on the go?

Samtosha (contentment) is a quality, a feeling, and a way of being with all experience—both positive and negative. Soften the struggle. Yoga asana and pranayama are useful tools for cultivating samtosha. Not only do we usually feel better after practice, but we can actually measure the grip of our restlessness or striving in the quality of our day-to-day practice. Cultivate contentment and let your heart bask in its own goodness, which is always enough.

JR

221.

To build character do something for no other reason than its difficulty.

WILLIAM JAMES

222.

Brahma and the other Devas were always engaged in the exercise of pranayama, and, by means of it, got rid of the fear of death. Therefore, one should practice pranayama regularly.

So long as the breath is restrained in the body, so long as the mind is undisturbed, and so long as the gaze is fixed between the eyebrows, there is no fear of Death.

HATHA YOGA PRADIPIKA

223.

My life when young was like a flower—a flower that loosens a petal or two from her abundance and never feels the loss when the spring breeze comes to beg at her door.

Now at the end of youth my life is like a fruit, having nothing to spare, and waiting to offer herself completely with her full burden of sweetness.

RABINDRANATH TAGORE

224.

The first question I ask myself when something
doesn't seem to be beautiful is why do I
think it's not beautiful. And very shortly
you discover that there is no reason.

JOHN CAGE

225.

DELICIOUS BREATH

Delicious breath blows through this body,
soft like crushed rose petal dust.
Transparent bones
land on mat.
Familiar dog folding forward and
back,

snake the spine around
this heart.
No tomorrow
no (to)night,
only now, delicious breath.

JR

226.

PRAYER FOR WELL-BEING

Sarve Bhavantu Sukhinah
Sarve Santu Niramaya
Sarve Bhadrani Pashyantu
Ma Kashchit Dukha Bhag Bhave

Om Shanti Shanti Shanti

May all be happy
May all be without suffering

May all think well of one another
May one's destiny be free from sorrow

JR

227.

SENSITIZE

Intelligently practiced, yoga develops one's sensitivity. It acts as a bridge to awareness and understanding of self and others. We must be careful not to use the practices as a way to numb ourselves in an obsessive or addictive way. Ideally, yoga helps us confront our difficulties without denying that they exist. On the other hand, if we become attached to the pleasure and bliss generated from intense yoga, we might get caught in the trap of seeking after these experiences. Better to enjoy our practice and move on: to drop into that place of goodness and peace in a single breath. Then we will stand free within yoga, not dependent upon it.

JR

228.

The quality of forgiveness that burns up all things except beauty is the quality of love. This love is that which removes the boundaries between self and self. When there is no longer a this-self and that-self, there can no longer be pain or separation. This brings about pure forgiveness—not something mental, not a changed attitude of mind, but a changed attitude of heart.

MURSHID SAMUEL LEWIS

229.

It has been my experience as a teacher that for most human beings, generally speaking, simply hearing the teaching is not enough. Usually they do need to have some kind of experience that makes the meaning of the words obvious in a very direct, experiential way. And then the person says, "Oh, my goodness, now

I understand! I've heard this for so many years, but now I recognize the truth of it."

ANDREW COHEN

230.

Whatever you do may seem insignificant, but it is most important that you do it.

GANDHI

231.

Be careful, very careful about organizations. Yoga cannot be organized, must not be organized. Organizations kill work. Love is everywhere, in everything, *is* everything. But if you confine it, enclose it in a box or in a definite place, it disappears. . . .

VANDA SCARAVELLI

232.

For the wonderful thing is that the body is not and never will be a machine, no matter how much we treat it as such, and, therefore, body movement is not and never will be mechanical—it is always and forever expressive, simply because it is human.

MARY STARKS WHITEHOUSE

233.

Heightened states of consciousness may arise from our experiments with yoga but if we chase after these states they become one more spoke on the wheel of *samsara*. Let them come and go without attachment and you will avoid disappointment.

JR

234.

If you conceptualize this teaching for your intellectual entertainment and do not let it act in your life, you will stumble and fall like a blind man.

YOGA VASISHTA

235.

[Non-attachment] should never be thought of as an austerity, a kind of self-torture, something grim and painful . . . And as we progress and gain increasing self-mastery, we shall see that we are renouncing nothing that we really need or want, we are only freeing ourselves from imaginary needs and desires.

SWAMI PRABHAVANANDA AND
CHRISTOPHER ISHERWOOD

236.

SRI LAKSHMI

The embodiment of the great mother goddess, the much beloved and honored Sri Lakshmi, finds a special place in the hearts of millions of devotees. Those who take refuge in her benefit from her awesome benevolence and compassion.

Lakshmi reigns in all matters pertaining to health, love, relationships, and wealth. She and her companion Vishnu sustain the cosmic order. She sits in the lotus pose (padmasana) upon a bed of lotus blossoms whose bowl-like shape resembles a womb. Surrounded by these flowers (symbols of fertility and creative energy), her lower hand forms the mudra of protection while the upper hand bestows blessings and gifts. Coins pour from the center of her palm in a gesture of generosity and abundance. Lakshmi's red or pink garments symbolize the loving heart. Meditate upon her and you will find love and many riches.

Practice
Visualize Sri Lakshmi and bring her into your heart. Meditate upon her. Repeat her name.

Gifts of Lakshmi
Health, love, abundance, relationship, mothering.

JR

237.

THE RUNGS OF LOVE

At first one loves only when one is loved in return.
Further on, one loves even if one is not loved but one
    still wants one's love to be
accepted. And finally one loves purely and simply with-
    out any other need or joy than
that of loving.

THE MOTHER

238.

The world is so you have something to stand on.

RUTH KRAUSS

239.

BINDU

The *bindu* represents the goddess Devi as the mother of creation. This small dot that sits inside the tip of the downward pointing triangle (*yoni* symbol) and on the space between the eyebrows of Hindu women represents the cosmos in the seed state of potentiality. On the island of Bali, grains of rice are fixed onto the third eye with water during religious ceremonies, literally acting as reminders of the "seed state."

Practice

You can use the *bindu* to visualize the perineum while working with *mulabandha* in sitting poses. All the energy inside the *yoni* triangle is channeled into this point and then gathered inward and upward. This visualization can be useful for women to strengthen the inner body and pelvic-floor muscles.

JR

240.

Unfortunately, to most people, enlightenment is like an old MGM production. They think it has to have all kinds of drama, stage settings, and a million other things. This is ridiculous. In reality, it is a great, great simplicity. It has to do with sitting inside of yourself and sensing the peace, quiet, and simplicity of a situation. It doesn't mean you don't see and experience life; it doesn't mean that you can't be alive, but you don't act out of your need for anything—you are free. And as you remain in this state, quietly, without drama, it becomes a fine flow—a very rich and simple flow.

SWAMI RUDRANANDA

241.

She who was burnt by the fire of Yoga
was born again in the Himalayas,
As she has the colour of the conch,
the Jasmine and the moon, she is called
"Gauri." May that Devi the destroyer of the pride of the
Kali age grant me pardon.

THE DEVI PURANA (PUPUL JAYAKAR)

242.

Take any one thing. What you don't know about it is always larger
than what you know.

SWAMI DAYANANDA SARASWATI

243.

PRANA AND THE NADIS

Prana animates the body. Often called "life force," it directs the energy of the universe, including our physical world and our thoughts. When prana does not flow we feel lifeless, stagnant, and confused. The *nadis,* or subtle nerve channels in the body (there are 72,000), allow prana to flow into the body. The three major *nadis* are *ida* (left side/lunar/feminine), *pingala* (right side/solar/masculine), and *sushumna* (center channel inside the spinal cord). The *nadis* are described eloquently in the "Siva Samhita." Directing the flow of prana into *sushumna* brings a state of optimum health and integration.

Yoga asanas open the nadis, and pranayama (yogic breathing) clears them of debris so that prana, or life force, can flow easily. The breath itself is our closest ally to prana. In order for breath to flow, the body must be available to the subtle chemistry of both.

Practice
Study pranayama with a competent teacher.

Balance the solar and lunar channels through the practice of *nadi shodhana* (*nadi* cleansing) and other breathing teachniques.

JR

244.

The ancient Vedic tradition of eating food with the hands is derived from mudra practice. Gathering the fingertips of the right hand as they touch the food stimulates the five elements and invites the fire of digestion to bring forth its digestive juices. In Vedic thought, the right hand beckons the solar energy of the body. The left hand (used for cleaning the body) beckons the lunar energy of the universe, inviting energy of completion or closure of the body. The *sadhana* of feeding yourself from hand to mouth enhances your vital memory and inner balance.

BRI MAYA TIWARI

245.

YOGA MUDRA

Mudras (seals) contain energy to create potent spiritual vehicles shaped from the body and breath. In yoga, dance, and other sacred arts mudras emulate the manifestations of various deities. In *anjali mudra,* with the palms sealed together to form the symbol of prayer, the gesture connects the aspirant to the divine within or to the personal deity called the *ishta devata.*

Many sculptures, wood carvings, and paintings from Asia illustrate the different gods and goddesses using hand mudras in devotional practice. In creating these images, artists themselves are engaged in yoga practices dedicated to representing the sacred play of life—*lila.*

Practice

Sit in the lotus or any other sustainable position. Place one hand lightly on each knee. Place both forefingers and both thumbs together and cup the palms upward. The connection of the thumb and forefinger keeps prana in the body and aids concentration. If your fingers should seperate, this signals that the mind needs to refocus. The circle captured in this gesture signifies the circle of life.

246.

OM Tryambakam yajamahe
Sugandhim pushti vardanam
Urvarukamiva bhandhanan
Mrityor mokshiya ma amritat-a

OM
We worship the three-eyed Lord Shiva who is full of
    sweet fragrance
And who nourishes all beings.
May he liberate me from bondage,
Just as the ripe cucumber is freed from its vine.
Let us not turn away from liberation.

MAHA MRITYUNJAYA MANTRA

247.

I don't know why it is we are in such a hurry to get up when we fall down. You might think we would lie there and rest a while.

MAX EASTMAN

248.

USTRASANA—CAMEL POSE

In the camel pose back bend, the heart center opens. Old fears may get stirred up as the upper body pours back over the legs, causing certain restrictions in the flow of breath and energy. For some, this pose seems to herald endless opening into the layers of the body and the possibility for true awakening.

Camel completely reverses our everyday posture by pulling the shoulders and back into a graceful arc, reminding us to look beneath the apparent nature of things. The camel guides us through the often bumpy terrain of back bends, cultivating patience and discernment. Through embodiment of this mysterious desert animal we come in contact with our own mystery. Like the camel, we may discover large reserves of energy and potential coming from within. The camel reminds us to replenish when our inner resources run low.

JR

249.

Yoga has been called a "fountain of youth" because it brings health and vitality, but this is a misnomer. The search for a fountain of youth, whether through magic, drugs, or techniques, indicates a resistance to the aging process. I prefer to call yoga a "fountain of life." Aging is inevitable. Yoga allows you to approach it awarely as a transformative process that can bring growth and new depths with maturation. Resisting aging is actually resisting transformation and growth. Paradoxically, the resistance to aging, which includes holding on to old, inappropriate ways of living, exacerbates the very aging process you fear.

JOEL KRAMER

250.

ALTERNATIVE YOGA *SADHANAS*

In the West, Hatha Yoga (primarily the body postures and breathing) tends to dominate our idea of yoga. But many other methods and practices (*sadhanas*) can bring us to a state of yoga. Simple daily tasks like gardening and cooking can become *sadhana* if performed with awareness and without attachment to outcome. Art is well suited to *sadhana*. Painting, writing, singing, and dancing can become sacred offerings. A useful way to turn creative endeavors into *sadhana* is to include them in your existing yoga practice. For example, after you finish asana, move into another form of practice. You may find that creative blocks vanish and that your art blossoms. Make sure that you frame the beginning and end of your practice with intentional focus using sound, silence, or mudras.

JR

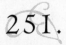

251.

Better indeed is knowledge than mechanical practice (of religious ritual). Better than knowledge is meditation. But better still is surrender of attachment to results (of one's actions), because there follows immediate peace.

BHAGAVAD GITA 12:12

252.

... the mind makes an effort. This did not come naturally, did it? ... It is very, very hard. Some "one" made a very hard effort. And those efforts resulted in a certain state of mind. ... Make any physical experiment or a chemical experiment. It is very clear, and this is the same in Yoga. Do step one, step two, step three, step four, step five. Ultimately, if all the earlier steps are done, a specific final result must come. But it is all still in phenomenality.

That is why Maharaj used to say, you may go into samadhi for ten minutes, you may go into samadhi for ten days, you may go into samadhi for ten years, you may go into samadhi for one hundred years, but you must come back where you left. Therefore it has no value.

RAMESH BALSEKAR

253.

For monogamy may be the best way for the body, but the soul that loves God in men dwells here always as the boundless and ecstatic polygamist; yet all the time—that is the secret—it is in love with only one being.

SRI AUROBINDO

254.

BUDDHI

Buddhi belongs to that part of the mind which acts as pure aware intelligence. *Buddhi* describes our ability for discernment and discrimination and is Buddhalike in nature. The *buddhi* expresses itself as the intuitive mind that awakens to truth. Clear as crystal, *buddhi* both supports and contains the *purusha*. This intelligence animates the universe.

JR

255.

HOME

Experience has shown me that everything seems to flow well after yoga and meditation practice. Connecting to my breath, moving through skin, I traverse muscle and bone and wash up on the shores of my own being. I find home.

JR

256.

Child, how happy you are sitting in the dust, playing
    with a broken twig all the morning.
I smile at your play with that little bit of a broken twig.
I am busy with my accounts, adding up figures by the
    hour.
Perhaps you glance at me and think, "What a stupid
    game to spoil your morning with!"

Child, I have forgotten the art of being absorbed in
    sticks and mud-pies.
I seek out costly playthings, and gather lumps of gold
    and silver.
With whatever you find you create your glad games, I
    spend both my time and my
strength over things I never can obtain. In my frail canoe
    I struggle to cross the sea of
desire, and forget that I too am playing a game.

RABINDRANATH TAGORE

257.

Love takes off masks that we fear we cannot live without and
know we cannot live within.

JAMES BALDWIN

258.

RHYTHM

Like music, yoga has rhythm. In your own practice this rhythm should be personal and specific to you. Often we get out of synch with our true nature. The food we eat, the work we do, and the people we share our lives with all affect our rhythm. In yoga practice the pace of your movement should ideally be performed to the rhythm of your breath. This may change from practice to practice.

Practice

　-Notice the state of your mind and how this influences
　 the pace of your practice.
　-Sustain a posture for many breaths. How does this feel?
　 What effect does this have on your mind?

JR

259.

In Tibetan the word for body is *lu*, which means "something you leave behind," like baggage. Each time we say "lu" it reminds us that we are only travelers, taking temporary refuge in this life and this body. So in Tibet people did not distract themselves by spending all their time trying to make their external circumstances more comfortable. They were satisfied if they had enough to eat, clothes on their backs, and a roof over their heads. Going on as we do, obsessively trying to improve our conditions, can become an end in itself and a pointless distraction. Would anyone in their right mind think of fastidiously redecorating their hotel room every time they booked into one?

SOGYAL RINPOCHE

260.

PLOWING THE SHOULDERS

Upside down. Fresh vistas.
Child's mind.
Flying backward legs over head,
I see life from a bug's-eye view and the sky looms large.
Firm base in the shoulders, spine long, fluids flowing swiftly
    through my cavernous body this
    way and that.
Liver, spleen, kidneys, stomach, intestines jostle for my
    attention.
Legs relieved of their usual burden, no longer have to hold
    me up. Now my shoulders get this
    privilege and my heart delights.

JR

261.

Persevering practice is the effort to attain and maintain the state of mental peace. Such a practice is firmly established only if one engages in it seriously and respectfully over a long and uninterrupted period.

YOGA SUTRA OF PATANJALI I:13–14

262.

I was walking along a little road through a hilly landscape; the sun was shining and I had a wide view in all directions. Then I came to a small wayside chapel. The door was ajar, and I went in. To my surprise there was no image of the Virgin on the altar, and no crucifix either, but only a wonderful flower arrangement. But then I saw that on the floor in front of the altar, facing *me*, sat a yogi—in lotus position, in deep meditation. When I looked at him more closely, I realized that he had *my* face. I started in profound fright, and awoke with the thought: "Aha, so he is the one who is meditating me. He has a dream, and I am it." I knew that when he awakened, I would no longer be.

C. G. JUNG

263.

Do not go to the garden of flowers!
  O Friend! go not there;
  In your body is the garden of flowers.
  Take your seat on the thousand petals of the lotus,
  And there gaze on the Infinite Beauty.

KABIR

264.

HATHA YOGA AND THE *NADIS*

Hatha Yoga includes the physical practices of body and breath. On another level, Hatha Yoga works with the subtle body of the *nadis* and chakras. Hatha derives from *ha* (the cool of the moon) and *tha* (the heat of the sun). *Ha* is connected to the *ida nadi* (lunar or left channel) and *tha* to the *pingala nadi* (solar or right channel). The central channel is called the *sushumna nadi.* Joining the moon and the sun together in *sushumna* so that the energy of prana can flow through this central axis is the goal of Hatha Yoga. This happens through physical practices of asana and pranayama. A well-crafted practice results in the subtle energies flowing freely.

Practice
As you practice asana and pranayama do you notice where energy constricts in the physical body and where it flows?

Turn your mind inward moving past the muscles, bones, and joints into the traveling currents of energy.

JR

265.

Clay-gods dissolve in the water,
Stone-gods break into pieces,
Metal-gods melt in the furnace,
Wooden-gods become ashes in the fire,
But the real One alone lives forever.

WISE SAYING

266.

Of (these) non-Vedic Saivas, the most important to art and literature were the Natha Jogis. The founder of this order was Gorakhanatha, a mysterious hero-figure, a magician, a Rasasiddha, and the founder of Hatha Yoga. It is from the orginal Hatha Yoga treatise of Gorakhanatha that the yogic images of the lotus and the chakras, with their colours, sounds and numbers, and also abstract visualizations of yogic phenomena, has its origin.

From Gorakhanatha also originate the imagery of the Kundalini, the dormant energy of yoga, asleep, coiled like a serpent at the base of the spine, as does the terminology of the *yoni*, the female generative organ, the "eye of love."

PUPUL JAYAKAR

267.

There is that ancient tree, whose roots grow upward and whose branches grow downward—that indeed is called the Bright, that is called Brahman, that alone is called the Immortal. All worlds are contained in it, and no one goes beyond. This is that.

KATHA UPANISHAD

268.

THE ART OF BREATHING

Breath animates the body and connects us to *purusha* (the spiritual principle). In yoga, the conscious control of the breath is known as pranayama, from *pran* (energy) and *yama* (restraint). When we breathe consciously light fills us and all circuits run more efficiently. Then the scattered mind draws into itself—revealing *Atman*.

Practice

- Integrate the breath movement with the body movement.
- Incorporate a sitting practice with pranayama into your other practices.
- Study pranayama with a teacher.
- Lengthen the exhale.
- Pause between inhale and exhale and between exhale and inhale.

JR

269.

Yoga is the dis-identification with the fluctuations of the mind.

JR

270.

Yoga is a harmony. Not for him who eats too much, or for him who eats too little; not for him who sleeps too little, or for him who sleeps too much.

BHAGAVAD GITA 6:16

271.

Weep at least once to see God.

SRI RAMAKRISHNA

272.

Understand that the socially imposed desires, such as the desire for God or "the desire for desire less-ness," dissociate us from the real movement of life and are not helpful. We don't take action in regard to real desire: we do not let the energy through and allow the natural wonder of relationship to do the yoga. In fact, free participation in the natural functions of life affirms our direct identity with that which is great.

MARK WHITWELL

273.

Meditation isn't to disappear into the light. Meditation is to see all of what we are.

STEPHEN LEVINE

274.

THE *GUNAS*

According to yoga, all life is composed of three elements. Known as the *gunas*, these elements have a specific quality: *Tamas*/inertia, *rajas*/activity, and *sattva*/harmony. At any given moment one *guna* will dominate, yet the three *gunas* constantly transform into each other. Becoming too attached to any one state creates imbalance. Even *sattva*, the state of perfection, cannot be maintained indefinitely.

Each *guna* has a quality of mind associated with it. *Tamas* generates little energy and makes it hard to get going. A heavy, foggy mind has a tamasic quality. On the other hand, a mind dominated by *rajas* gets things done quickly, but is often shadowed by hyperactivity. The rajasic mind taken to an extreme can result in hypertension and stress. *Sattva*, the harmonious mind, sees things clearly and brings peace. Becoming aware of how the *gunas* operate within us will help sort out imbalances.

Practice

Observe your yoga practice. Do you tend to rush through the poses hoping to cram as many of them into your practice as possible? Do you often opt only for vigorous classes? This might indicate a dominance of *rajas*. Or maybe it takes you a long time to get going. Here you may tend toward *tamas*. What happens on the days when you feel wonderfully present and in balance? Do you chase after these "good" practice times and discount the other practices as unworthy?

Yoga is navigating the difficulty without judgment. Understanding that all practice efforts are worthwhile (even the ones that do not flow) leads to self-acceptance.

JR

275.

One who pervades
the great Universe
is seen by none
unless a man knows
the unfolding
of love.

CHANDIDAS

276.

SITTING MOVEMENT

Begin and complete each asana practice with a short or long sitting meditation. Notice if discomfort arises in the body/mind. If you become restless, try not to run away, but instead ask yourself who is restless? Let it run its course. If your discomfort with sitting becomes unbearable, start to move. (Use a breath and movement posture sequence or other movement that you know.) In what way does the discomfort change?

JR

277.

Dance then, Lalla, clothed but in the air:
Sing then, Lalla, clad but in the sky.
Air and sky: what garment is more fair?
"Cloth," said Custom—Doth that sanctify?

LALLA

278.

It is conceived of by him by whom It is not conceived of. He by whom It is conceived of, knows It not. It is not understood by those who (say they) understand It. It is understood by those who (say they) understand It not.

KENA UPANISHAD

279.

Even this practice of getting oneself fully conscious, and the sound AUM each marching into the other and getting telescoped in themselves one into the other, is in itself a severe training for the mind at concentration. The conscious superimpositions unfolded and again folded up, as explained above, is an equally all-absorbing occupation for the entire intellectual capacity in us, so that the true practitioner if he be sincere and regular, gains in a very short time an infinite amount of integration both in his mind and intellect.

SWAMI CHINMAYANANDA

280.

O servant, where dost thou seek Me?
Lo! I am beside thee.

I am neither in temple nor in mosque:
I am neither in Kaaba nor in Kailash:

Neither am I in rites and ceremonies,
nor in Yoga and renunciation.

If thou art a true seeker, thou shalt at once see Me:
thou shalt meet Me in a moment of time.

Kabir says, "O Sadhu! God is the breath of all breath."

KABIR

281.

In the midst of winter, I finally learned that there was in me an
invincible summer.

ALBERT CAMUS

282.

AHIMSA—NONVIOLENCE

One of the yamas and a guiding core principle of yoga, ahimsa is as vital to our practice as the standing poses or downward-facing dog. This attitude of nonviolence that we strive to cultivate in all of life brings us face-to-face with desire, anger, and memory. Practice nonviolence in all aspects of life: in thought, speech, and action. From the food you eat to the thoughts you consume cultivate ahimsa.

JR

283.

The ego is like a stick that seems to divide the water in two. It makes you feel that you are one and I am another. When the ego disappears in *samadhi* one realizes Brahman as one's own inner consciousness.

SRI RAMAKRISHNA

284.

When your understanding has passed beyond the thicket of delusions, there is nothing you need to learn from even the most sacred scripture.

BHAGAVAD GITA 2:52

285.

Today there is no longer a choice between violence and nonviolence. It is either nonviolence or nonexistence. I feel that we've got to look at this total thing anew and recognize that we must live together. That the whole world now it is one—not only geographically but it has to become one in terms of brotherly concern. Whether we live in America or Asia or Africa we are all tied in a single garment of destiny and whatever affects one directly, affects one indirectly.

DR. MARTIN LUTHER KING, JR.

286.

PARIGHASANA: THE GATEWAY

The gateway asana encourages transformation. Practice of this intense side stretch takes us beyond our daily lives, stretching our boundaries so that we can move past limitations. Kneeling with one leg firmly on the earth, parighasana teaches us how to remain grounded while reaching for our dreams. The arc of the body is a passageway between the earth and sky connecting the elements of nature that are present within us. Through yoga practice the gate within opens. Obstacles on our path dissolve and the spirit soars. In this posture the peripheries of the body/mind are expanded— taking us into new territory and into new consciousness.

Practice

-Where are the gateways in your own body?

-Which asanas help you to move and expand your sense of who you are?

-What territory needs to be explored?

JR

287.

In asana practice, each part of the body becomes an expression of the desire to realize God. The hands, fingers, feet, toes, and all the body parts express this yearning for the Divine.

SHARON GANNON AND DAVID LIFE

288.

Only when you put away the things of the mind, only when your heart is empty of the things of the mind, is there love. Then you will know what it is to love without separation, without distance, without time, without fear—and that is not reserved for the few. Love knows no hierarchy; there is only love. There are the many and the one, an exclusiveness, only when you do not love. When you love, there is neither the "you" nor the "me." In that state there is only a flame without smoke.

J. KRISHNAMURTI

289.

When you know you don't know it makes sense to ask. If you were to get lost while driving through an unfamiliar town, for example, you wouldn't hesitate to stop and either ask someone for directions or look at a map. It is the same here; however, instead of looking at an external map or asking someone else for directions, you ask inwardly, using your mind to commune with Infinite Mind. You ask the traffic helicopter. You talk to God. You ask inwardly to your Self—like a wave to the ocean, a cell to the brain, or a cloud to the sky. You ask the larger portion of you, the part that knows. You ask and listen and lo and behold . . . you find yourself knowing.

ERICH SCHIFFMANN

290.

KARMA YOGA

To know God is to serve others as if they were God.

SOURCE UNKNOWN

One of the branches on the tree of yoga, Karma Yoga refers to the Yoga of Action. Taking action—yet not being attached to the fruits of action—is a central theme of the *Bhagavad Gita*.

In practice, Karma Yoga has come to be associated with service. Mother Teresa devoted her life to serving the poor and destitute. Her path can be seen as a practice of Karma Yoga as she offered up her work to God and surrendered the results to this higher power. Donating time and energy to others is Karma Yoga.

JR

291.

If you can't feed a hundred people, then feed just one.

MOTHER TERESA

292.

Guru Brahma Guru Vishnu
Guru Devo Maheshwara
Guru Saksat Paramguru
Tasmai Sri Guruve Namah

Guru is Brahma, Guru is Vishnu,
Guru is Lord Shiva.
To that Guru,
The Highest Manifestation of Reality, I bow.

SANSKRIT MANTRA

293.

The teacher who walks in the shadow of the temple,
among his followers, gives not of his wisdom but rather
   of his faith
and his lovingness. If he is indeed wise he does not bid
   you enter the house of his wisdom
but rather leads you to the threshold of your own
   mind.

KAHLIL GIBRAN

294.

Truly there is no cause for you to be miserable and unhappy. You
yourself impose limitations on your own true nature of infinite
Being, and then weep that you are but a finite creature. Then you
take up this or that *sadhana* to transcend the non-existent limita-

tions. But if your *sadhana* itself assumes the existence of the limitations, how can it help you to transcend them?

SRI RAMANA MAHARSHI

295.

FAITH—*ISHVARAPRANIDHANA*

As we journey on the path of yoga, we may encounter all sorts of obstacles. Day after day, week after week, we come back to our mats and our bodies, to our breath and our prayers. This return can be seen as faith-in-action. Somewhere inside we believe that yoga will help us. Maybe it will heal our lower-back pain or depression or make us stronger, more flexible, and beautiful. Maybe it will bring us closer to God, Goddess, or to the source of our being. Called to play in different forms, we trust this process. We might not understand this faith, yet it informs our experience of yoga. When something greater than intellect and larger than the will or ego is at work, we have touched faith and experienced *ishvarapranidhana*, the spiritual principle in yoga.

JR

296.

Repeating the sacred syllable and pondering its meaning lead to its understanding. It is then that one understands the self and gradually clears inner obstacles.

YOGA SUTRA OF PATANJALI I:28–29

297.

Wanting and not wanting are both you.
The movement of wanting can never stop.
Wanting not to want is also a want.
The ending of want is death.

U. G. KRISHNAMURTI

298.

Through yoga we feel change as it occurs. We become both the
change and the witness to it.

JR

299.

Many go fishing all their lives without knowing that it is not fish they are after.

HENRY DAVID THOREAU

300.

Asana practice should be a harmonious experience, never a struggle. The manner of breathing into a wind instrument—a flute, for instance—can create either a grating screech or a melodious song. The body, too, is an instrument. If used skillfully, as in the unison of movement and breath, the resulting posture is a useful and harmonious experience. When performed with the graceful orchestration of all its parts, asana can become a music of the body, breath, and mind. Such music moves everything it touches.

A. G. MOHAN

301.

GARUDASANA—THE EAGLE

Garuda, the Hindu deity with a bird face and human body, is known as Lord of the Birds. The god Vishnu rides upon this winged creature who, with his eagle-like vision, sees far and wide. In yoga practice, this posture makes a human spiral out of the body. Both the arms and legs wrap around each other, creating a figure eight containing the life energy of the spiral within. Both outer and inner spirals need to be maintained in order to find the balance and integrity of the pose. Through this balance, we feel our natural radiance and affirmation for all of life.

Practice

By embodying this majestic bird in the pose of the eagle, we learn about freedom and balance. We begin to cultivate wisdom, compassion, and the intense visionary powers that flying high in the sky can bring.

JR

302.

LAUGHING AT
THE WORD TWO

Only
That Illumined
One
Who keeps
Seducing the formless into form
Had the charm to win my
Heart.
Only a perfect One
Who is always laughing at the word
Two
Can make you know
Of
Love.

HAFIZ

303.

Whether or not enlightenment is a plausible goal for us is a vital question for our lives. If it is possible for us to be open to attain such perfect enlightenment ourselves, our whole sense of meaning and our place in the universe immediately changes . . . Once we recognize the biological possibility of our evolving into beings of full understanding, we can begin to imagine ourselves as buddhas, awakened or enlightened beings.

ROBERT THURMAN

304.

Selfishness kills the soul; destroy it.
But take care that your altruism does not kill the souls of others.

SRI AUROBINDO

305.

One of the Sanskrit words for the cosmos is *jagat*, "the moving thing." In the Ayurvedic model the universe is declared to be eternal without beginning, continuously moving, periodically manifesting from a singularity and periodically resolving into un-manifestation, waxing and waning like the moon. A human being likewise begins from a zygote, a single cell containing all his or her potentialities, which explosively projects those potentialities into a physical form that, like the universe and its individual stars, grows and develops, reaches a stable plateau and then degenerates and dies.

The singularity that creates the cosmos is, like the zygote or the seed of a tree, the cause of the dualistic being it creates, which is the effect. In the words of my teacher, Vimalananda, "cause is effect concealed, and effect is cause revealed."

ROBERT SVOBODA

306.

All plants are our brothers and sisters.
They talk to us and if we listen,
We can hear them.

ARAPAHO PROVERB

307.

So Ham
Tat Twam Asi
Aham Brahmasmi

I am That.
Thou are That.
I am Brahman.

SANSKRIT MANTRA

308.

Do not kill the instinct of the body for the glory of the pose.

VANDA SCARAVELLI

309.

The body is the physical aspect of the personality and movement is the personality made visible.

MARY STARKS WHITEHOUSE

310.

Anything that happens in the present moment is necessary. So, if someone is doing meditation, I just say continue with your meditation. If you are doing yoga, continue with the yoga. The only thing is, if some change happens, not to have a feeling of guilt. Therefore, don't try to make any changes. Continue with your life and if some changes take place, accept them without a sense of guilt.

RAMESH BALSEKAR

311.

Never doubt that a small group of thoughtful, committed citizens can change the world. Indeed, it is the only thing that ever has.

MARGARET MEAD

312.

We must recognize the Mother in all her aspects. To the sages, the streams and rivers that flow in the Himalayas are the divinity of Dhari Devi, "Goddess of the Current." Himalayan peaks such as Badrinath and Kadarnath are also adored as her manifestation. The next time you stand in an open meadow, notice your mind shift as you watch the wind sweep through the grass. When you are in a rainstorm, listen to your heart pound with the pulse of the drops and rhythms of the water. This alignment with the forces of nature is a function of our *shakti*-prana, the breath of the Mother moving within you.

BRI MAYA TIWARI

313.

THE YOGA OF
NON-ATTACHMENT

For some yoga can become an obsession. Natural enthusiasm and commitment to yoga is very different from compulsion. Engage in a balanced, holistic practice. Approach yoga with non-attachment, and joy, and especially with love.

JR

314.

Don't grieve.
Anything you lose comes round in another form.
The child weaned from mother's milk
now drinks wine and honey mixed.

KABIR

315.

As the rivers flowing east and west
Merge in the sea and become one with it,
Forgetting they were ever separate rivers,
So do all creatures lose their separateness
When they merge at last into pure Being.

CHANDOGYA UPANISHAD

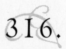

316.

I still miss those I loved who are no longer with me but I find I am grateful for having loved them. The gratitude has finally conquered the loss.

RITA MAE BROWN

317.

When the mind is not turned outward it reflects consciousness itself.

YOGA SUTRA OF PATANJALI 4:22

318.

This world is all attachment. Yet you get worried because you are attached.

NEEM KAROLI BABA

319.

BALANCE

Careful construction of your Hatha Yoga practice is like creating a tasty meal with all the right spices. The food is satisfying when the spices are in balance. So, too, in creating a yoga practice that leads to a harmonious mind. On some days, you might require more movement with lots of variety, while on others, your system may need more stillness. Tune in to your needs and over time you will be able to observe the three *gunas* intertwining and acting within you as one.

JR

320.

Love truth, but pardon error.

VOLTAIRE

321.

YOGA AS PRAYER

Dedicate your practice to something meaningful and true. Initiate your practice from this place and let it become a prayer of spontaneous movement and joy. Sing or chant as you move and don't be afraid to take risks. Explore the uncharted seas of your body. Be the love that you seek. Let your practice be the prayer itself, your body the temple.

JR

322.

Let him close the ears with his thumbs, the eyes with index fingers, the nostril with the middle fingers, and with the remaining four fingers let him press together the upper and lower lips. The Yogi, by having thus firmly confined the air, sees his soul in the shape of light.

SIVA SAMHITA

323.

ALL LIFE IS YOGA

SRI AUROBINDO

Once we understand that all life is yoga, we give up the search. We become less attached to whether we experience pleasure or pain, knowing that both positive and negative states spring from the same source. When we recognize that everything is yoga, we stop having preferences that keep us bound in endless cycles of seeking.

JR

324.

Is there a difference between pure consciousness and utter void? Even if there is, it is impossible to put it into words.

YOGA VASISTHA

325.

JNANA YOGA

Also known as the Yoga of Wisdom, Jnana Yoga uses the mind (*manas*) and discriminating intelligence (*buddhi*). Devotion to this sacred principle comes through such channels as the study of sacred texts, discussion of important themes with a reliable teacher, or regular meditation. Jnana Yoga merges the heart and mind into powerful practice.

JR

326.

Wanting You—I lost the walls of me—
dropped my scales of petal and thorn
and into the empty room I ran
sweet and wild like a child.

JONATHAN LEWIS

327.

Come out into the broad light of day, come out from the little narrow paths, for how can the infinite soul rest content to live and die in small ruts? Come out into the universe of Light. Everything in the universe is yours, stretch out your arms and embrace it with love. If you ever felt you wanted to do that, you have felt God.

SWAMI VIVEKANANDA

328.

VINYASA

The great yoga adept Sri T. Krishnamacharya developed the concept of *vinyasa*. While commonly thought to mean a strong flow of postures choreographed in a predetermined series, *vinyasa* encompasses more than "flow." *Vinyasa* links the poses in an intentional and progressive sequence in order to lead the practitioner from his current place toward a particular posture and state of mind. *Vinyasa* links the body to the breath and the breath to the mind in a seamless unobstructed flow that carries over into daily life and helps us tune in to the flow of universal energy.

JR

329.

Time in the form of night and day is made by the sun and moon. That the Sushumna devours this time (death) is a great secret.

HATHA YOGA PRADIPIKA

330.

KUNDALINI

Kundalini energy, represented by a serpent with its tail in its mouth, contains the divine feminine energy known as *shakti*. In most of us she lies dormant, coiled around the *sushumna nadi*, near the base of the spine. She awaits until awakened by spiritual *tapas* or spontaneous opening to join in union with pure consciousness. Her journey through the chakras clears obstructions in these areas. As she uncoils and rises up, the yogi's consciousness also rises. If it rises enough, intense lucidity, altered consciousness, or enlightenment may occur.

On a more earthly level, we can understand the workings of *kundalini* from a simple practice of asana, pranayama, and meditation. In order for *kundalini* to move, each chakra must be open. Yoga practices that open and purify the body release the *kundalini* energy.

JR

331.

He who sees all beings in his Self and his Self in all beings, he never suffers; because when he sees all creatures within his true Self, then jealousy, grief and hatred vanish. He alone can love.

ISAVASYA UPANISHAD

332.

There are no guarantees. From the viewpoint of fear, none are strong enough. From the viewpoint of love, none are necessary.

EMMANUEL

333.

CHILDREN AND YOGA

The great yogi of the twentieth century T. Krishnamacharya emphasized the importance of teaching yoga to children. Bonding with young children through the body and the imagination strengthens the relationship between adults and children. Children remind us to be spontaneous and playful with our practice, and infants remind us of our earliest movement origins and capabilities. They put us in touch with the pure joy and love of movement.

JR

334.

The symbols of the self arise in the depths of the body.

C. G. JUNG

335.

Our thoughts have been scattered, as it were, all over the mental field. Now we begin to collect them again and to direct them toward a single goal—knowledge of the *Atman*. As we do this we find ourselves becoming increasingly absorbed in the thought of what we are seeking. And so, at length, absorption merges into illumination, and the knowledge is ours.

CHRISTOPHER ISHERWOOD
AND SWAMI PRABHAVANANDA

336.

A sage partakes of sensuous pleasures as they occur with a detached mind and does not become addicted to desire.

GOPALA UTTARA TAPINI UPANISHAD

337.

DISCIPLE: But I have heard it said by a Saint that his spiritual experience is felt at the place between the eyebrows.

RAMANA: As I said previously that is the ultimate and perfect Realization which transcends subject-object relation. When that is achieved, it does not matter where the spiritual experience is felt.

DISCIPLE: But the question is which is the correct view of the two, namely, (1) that the centre of spiritual experience is the place between the eyebrows, (2) that it is the Heart.

RAMANA: For purposes of practice concentrate between the eyebrows; it would then be *bhavana* or imaginative contemplation of the mind; whereas the supreme state of *Anubhava* or Realization, with which you become wholly identified and in which your individuality is completely dissolved, transcends the mind. Then, there can be no objectified centre to be experienced by you as a subject distinct and separate from it.

SRI RAMANA MAHARSHI

338.

Another very common story that circulates in New Age circles leads to the conclusion that when you are experiencing some particular trouble in the human predicament, God is testing you, or that this is a new lesson, or maybe it is to strengthen your resolve and your will power. Friends, Source does not need any lessons or testing. It already knows it all. This is a dream about limitation. The dream is scheduled to end. No time has actually elapsed. No damage has been done. No lessons learned. Nobody died, because they were never born!

SATYAM NADEEN

339.

He sees himself in the heart of all beings and he sees all beings in his heart. This is the vision of the Yogi of harmony, a vision which is ever one.

And when he sees me in all and he sees all in me, then I never leave him and he never leaves me.

He who in this oneness of love, loves me in whatever he sees, wherever this man may live, in truth this man lives in me.

BHAGAVAD GITA 6:29–31

340.

EFFORTLESS EFFORT

Dropping into asana, breath and meditation as an integral part of everyday life makes yoga a natural fluid process. Effortless effort. No need to feel proud about the time we set aside for yoga. Pride in our practice builds up the ego. Conversely, if we somehow fail to practice there is no guilt, no remorse, and no inner critic. We simply make time for practice the next day and begin anew.

JR

341.

It is not necessary to meet your guru on the physical plane. The guru is not external.

NEEM KAROLI BABA

342.

Mind is the seed, pranayama the soil, dispassion the water. Out of these three grows the tree that fulfills all wishes.

HATHA YOGA PRADIPIKA

343.

The masters say: "If you create an auspicious condition in your body and your environment, then meditation and realization will automatically arise." Talk about posture is not esoteric pedantry; the whole point of assuming a correct posture is to create a more inspiring environment for meditation, for the awakening of Rigpa. There is a connection between the posture of the body and the attitude of the mind. Mind and body are interrelated, and meditation arises naturally once your posture and attitude are inspired.

SOGYAL RINPOCHE

344.

When the sage of silence, the Muni, closes the doors of his soul and, resting his inner gaze between the eyebrows, keeps peaceful and even the ebbing and flowing of breath;

and with life and mind and reason in harmony, and with desire and fear and wrath gone, keeps silent his soul before final freedom, he in truth has attained final freedom.

BHAGAVAD GITA 5:28–29

345.

The art of being wise is the art of knowing what to overlook.

WILLIAM JAMES

346.

This self-knowledge is not gained by explanations and descriptions, nor by the instructions of others. At all times, everything is known only by direct experience.

YOGA VASISTHA

347.

Soul, why hast thou become beggar? Thrice-wretched, knowing nought? In search of the wealth that passes, thou art wandering from land to land. That which thou desirest, which thou lovest, seest thou not within thine home? Soul, if thou but quit thyself like mind, thou shalt come to union. When worship comes easy and natural as thy breath, then death's poison will have no power upon thee. The jewels and the wealth thy teachers have given, bind them fast to thee. This is the request of poor Ramaprasad, who hopes to touch the Feet that banish fear.

RAMPRASAD SEN

348.

MALASANA: SQUATTING POSES

This powerful asana is part of everyday life for many millions of men and women who assume the position for the daily activities of cooking, eating, chatting, and elimination. In many cultures, even very elderly people can squat with comfort and ease. In industrial cultures, we have lost our connection to this powerful seat. Physiologically, squats aid digestion and lengthen the muscles of the back, hips, and groin.

In yoga, we can use squats to ground and connect to the forces of the earth. This is a pose of immanence rooted to the feminine energy of creation and birth. The original birthing position, the squat helps pregnant women learn to open and release.

Squats take us inside ourselves and keep us rooted to life and all its wonders. Working with gravity by letting the pose unfold moment by moment, we let go of all that binds us physically and emotionally.

JR

349.

Man's perceptions are not bound by organs of perception; he perceives more than sense (tho' ever so acute) can discover.

WILLIAM BLAKE

350.

Yoga is not a self-improvement program. Let go of ideas of perfection and come into yourself just as you are.

JR

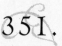

351.

Every man is more than just himself; he also represents the unique, the very special and always significant and remarkable point at which the world's phenomena intersect, only once in this way and never again.

HERMANN HESSE

352.

Who would stand in the scorching heat of the sun, when there is the cool shade of a tree? This cool shade can only be found in solitude which is a state of mind. True solitude is not, therefore, an isolation from the rest.

SWAMI NIRMALANANDA

353.

We read, we try to understand, to explain, we try to know. But a single minute of true experience teaches us more than millions of words and hundreds of explanations.

THE MOTHER

354.

UTTIHITA TRIKONASANA— TRIANGLE POSE

The goddess of renowned form assumes, in time of protection, the form of a straight line; in time of destruction she takes the form of a circle, and for creation she takes on the brilliant appearance of a triangle.

KAMAKALA-CHIDVALLI

The triangle has long been associated with the divine feminine in Indian culture, religion, and art. The three lines that make up a triangle form the basis of the *yantra*. As a yoga pose, the triangle becomes the embodied representation of the mystery of the universe and creation. The triangle is worshiped in the form of the *yoni* and is given a feminine attribute. Literally, the *yoni* (vulva) is the abode of birth and of cosmic creation. When practicing trikonasana, we make this symbol alive by allowing the earth energy to rise first through the feet and then through the legs (two points of the triangle). We then deliver the earth to the sky in the third point of the triangle symbolized by the upward stretched arm and supported by the lower lengthened arm.

The *yoni*, represented as a downward-pointing triangle, contains a circle reduced to a small red dot in its center known as a *bindu*. The *bindu* contains the essence of the universe and is itself enclosed by the triangle. Tri (three) is the sacred number of the three *gunas*, known as *sattva*, *rajas*, and *tamas*, and the three *doshas* known as *vata*, *pitta*, and *kapha*. Three is the cycle of universal energy: creation, preservation, and destruction. Learning to balance the three constituents of nature develops individual and universal harmony. Through active meditation upon the triangle we create harmonious living.

JR

355.

As long as the Prana does not enter and flow in the middle channel and the *vindu* does not become firm by the control of the movements of the Prana; as long as the mind does not assume the form of Brahma without any effort in contemplation, so long all the talk of knowledge and wisdom is merely the nonsensical babbling of a mad man.

HATHA YOGA PRADIPIKA

356.

Even as a mirror stained by dust shines brightly when it has been cleaned, so the embodied one when he had seen the (real) nature of the Self becomes integrated, of fulfilled purpose and freed from sorrow.

SVETASVATARA UPANISHAD

357.

Everything continues to rise moment to moment—the entire Kosmos continues to arise moment to moment—but there is nobody watching the display, a spontaneous and luminous gesture of great perfection. The pure Emptiness of the Witness turns out to be one with every Form that is witnessed, and that is one of the basic meanings of "non-duality."

KEN WILBER

358.

DHANURASANA — BOW

The bow acts as a link to the divine. As the hands clasp the feet, unity is born from the limbs. One of the aims of yoga practice is to "yoke" or to bring the physical, mental, emotional, and energetic levels into wholeness. Bow exemplifies the qualities that are needed for completion: openness, flexibility, faith, courage, and strength. Patanjali tells us that in practice, postures should be both firm and soft. These qualities are evident in this deep back bend that relies on the belly for balance. Bow invites us through the gate of the body to ponder the treasures held within.

JR

All illustrations are inadequate and truth is beyond words.

YOGA VASISTHA

360.

No mortal lives by the breath that goes up and by the breath that goes down. We live by another, in whom these two repose.

KATHA UPANISHAD

361.

Your job will be that of yielding to the flow. Traditionally, this has been called "surrender." It is the active choice for "Thy will be done." It is the most intelligent, fulfilling thing to do. You surrender your best sense of what to do or not do, and instead trust in the flow of Being. This is when yoga becomes more than practice and practices—and becomes your way of life. Then you realize there is no such thing as practice! Never was. There is only the real thing, ever—and always.

ERIC SCHIFFMANN

362.

Those who in the devotion of Yoga rest all their soul ever on me, very soon come unto me.

BHAGAVAD GITA 8:14

363.

This world is not conclusion;
A sequel stands beyond.
Invisible as music,
But positive as sound.

EMILY DICKINSON

364.

ELEMENTS

I am the breath that moves the wind in the sky,
The body that transforms into earth's rich soil.
I am the heat that burns in the fire of devotion.
I am the source that makes the rain pour and the rivers flow.
I am the ethereal space between thoughts, between breaths.
I am the Mother of all children, the Father of all ages.
I am male and female both together.
I am You in this body.
You are me, in mine.

JR

365.

Om! This syllable is the whole world.
The past, the present, the future—everything is just the word *Om*.

MANDUKYA UPANISHAD

GLOSSARY

Ahimsa	One of the yamas meaning nonharming. This concept of nonviolence is an integral foundation of all yoga.
Amrita	Nectar of immortality, drunk by the Gods
Anandamayima, Sri	One of the great female gurus, saints of India
Anandatandava	Eternal bliss
Ananta	Endless. The Infinite. Cosmic serpent.
Ajna chakra	One of seven major energy centers in the human body located in the space between the eyebrows. Also known as the "third eye" and seat of wisdom.
Apana-vayu	One of the principle pranas, known as the downward breath, or eliminating breath
Asana	Literally means the seat. Body postures assumed in yoga practice.
Ashtanga	Patanjali's Yoga: the Eight-Limbed Path
Atman	The true self—that which is eternal

Aurobindo, Sri	The founder of Integral Yoga. One of the most important contemporary Indian sages who developed a spiritual yoga for the evolution of modern consciousness. The author of hundreds of books on Yoga. He developed his system with his spiritual partner, The Mother.
Avidya	One of the *klesas,* meaning false understanding, misapprehension
Ayurveda	An ancient Indian healing art developed from the Vedas
Bandha	An internal technique in Hatha Yoga that locks the energy of *prana* in the body
Bhagavad Gita	Also known as *The Song of God.* The great Indian text that is part of the larger epic called *The Mahabharata.* In the Gita, Arjuna learns yoga from the Lord Krishna.
Bhakti	The practice of devotional yoga
Bhava	An attitude of devotion
Bhavana	Meditation or visualization
Bija	Seed
Buddhi	Intellect. The discriminating faculty.

Chakra	An energy center known as a wheel. There are seven chakras, which lie along the spinal column.
Chela	Student
Dharma	One's moral duty and path
Guna	A quality of being that evokes a feeling in the mind. The *gunas* make up the qualities in the universe.
Guru	A teacher. Literally, one who dispels darkness and brings light.
Hafiz	This great Persian poet and Sufi master who wrote mystical poetry revealing the playful heart of spiritual genius
Hazrat Inayat Khan	An Indian Sufi master who brought the Sufi teachings to the West. Well known for his understanding of the mystical nature of sound and music.
Ishta devata	Chosen deity for devotional practices
Ishvara	The spiritual principle in Yoga. God. Source. Divine quality.
Ishvarapranidhana	Surrender to the spiritual. Faith as described in *The Yoga Sutras.*

Jalandhara-bandha	A Hatha Yoga technique that consists of nestling the chin into the throat chakra to prevent the *amrita* from moving downward. Chin lock.
Japa	The repetition of a mantra usually done with a rosary or beaded necklace
Kabir	Born a Muslim, later converted to Hinduism. He was one of the great poet saints of medieval India often associated with Sufism.
Kaivalya	Freedom and peace. The ultimate stage and state of yoga according to Patanjali.
Klesha	Affliction
Krishnamacharya	The father of modern yoga. A twentieth-century Indian yoga master, Krishnamacharya profoundly influenced yoga in both India and the West. His students included B. K. S. Iyengar, K. Pattabhi Jois, and his son T. V. K. Desikachar. He is considered to be the "teacher of teachers."
Kundalini	The serpent energy that awakens through the Hatha Yoga practice
Lalla	A bhakta and yogini in the Kashmiri Shaivism tradition. Famous for her mystical writings.
Mantra	A sacred syllable that often connotes a specific spiritual principle or deity

Mirabai	A mystic poet-saint of India—a bhakta. Her haunting songs to Lord Krishna are still sung throughout India today.
Moksha	Liberation. Final freedom.
The Mother	Originally from France, The Mother (Mère) was a great mystic of the twentieth century who, together with Sri Aurobindo, developed Integral Yoga.
Mudra	A symbolic seal—usually a gesture made with the hands or whole body that promotes concentration in yoga and dance postures.
Mukti	Total identification with God. Freedom or release from suffering.
Nad(a)	The yoga of sound
Nadis	Important channels in a yogi's subtle body. Irrigated *nadis* carry the flow of prana into the central or *sushumna nadi*. Likened to nerve centers. A focus of pranayama.
Nirvikalpa Samadhi	Pure supra-conscious ecstasy. A sustained state.
Niyama	Discipline. Relationship toward oneself.
Patanjali	The codifier of *The Yoga Sutras*. Thought to be an incarnation of Ananta, the cosmic serpent.

Prakriti	The universe manifest. Matter.
Prana	The life force that animates the body
Pranava	Referred to in *The Yoga Sutras* as the mystical sound OM
Pranayama	Extension of the breath. The various Hatha Yoga breathing practices.
Purusha	That which sees. The Perceiver.
Rasa	Has several meanings including: juice, essence, and taste. An important concept in Ayurveda.
Sadhana	Practice
Sahaja	That which is most natural
Samadhi	A state of realization. Enlightenment.
Samsara	The cycle of birth, death, and rebirth. Material existence.
Samskara	The mental patterns or grooves—our conditioning
Samtosha	Contentment
Shakti	Power. The feminine energy that is embodied in the Mother Goddess. A complementary force to Shiva. Shakti is also a goddess.

Siddha	One who has a special yogic gift or power
Soma	Like Amrita, a powerful ambrosial elixir of the gods thought to be traced to an actual herb or plant
Sushumna nadi	Central channel in the human body
Svadhyaya	Self-examination and understanding. Study of sacred texts
Tagore, Rabindranath	One of the great twentieth-century poets. Born in Bengal, India, and awarded the Nobel prize for literature.
Tapas	A rigorous spiritual practice that cleanses
Uddiyana-bandha	A Hatha Yoga technique known as the "upward lock" and performed by lifting the area of the navel upward to direct and contain the pranic flow
Upanishad	Mystical teachings of India. Also known as "approaches" from the root word *upa*, which means near, and *shad*, which means sit. Sit near the teacher and receive the sacred teachings.
Vairagya	Nonattachment
Vasana	Desire and the remnants left by desire in the mind

Vayu	Wind, or vital air, of which there are five: *prana, apana, samana, udana, and vyana*
The Vedas	Ancient books of spiritual wisdom from India
Veena	A wooden stringed instrument played by the goddess Saraswati
Vinyasa	A sequence of asanas linked to breath building to a goal that returns the practitioner to a new and perhaps transformed mental place
Yama	Disciplined attitude concerning how we relate to the world and others
Yantra	A sacred geometrical symbol in Indian art
Yogi	A practitioner of yoga
Yogini	A female adept, mendicant, goddess, or Hatha/ Tantra Yoga practitioner
Yoni	Vulva. Considered the site of all creation, and therefore it is honored and worshiped in Tantra Yoga and in the worship of the goddess.

REFERENCES

Actuelles-Ecrits Politiques, Albert Camus, Gallimard, Paris (reprint), 1977. (no. 281)

"Advaita 101: An Interview with Swami Dayananda Saraswati," Andrew Cohen in *What Is Enlightenment?* Issue 14, spring/summer 1998. (no. 229)

Advanced Course in Yogi Philosophy and Oriental Occultism, Yogi Ramacharaka, the Yogi Publication Society, Chicago, 1904. (nos. 60, 134)

Ageless Body, Timeless Mind: The Quantum Alternative to Growing Old, Deepak Chopra, M.D., Harmony Books, New York, 1993. (no. 186)

All Men Are Brothers—Autobiographical Reflections, Mahatma Gandhi (editor), Krishna Kripalani Continuum, New York, 1980. (no. 190)

Anandamayi, Life and Wisdom, Richard Lannoy, Element, London, 1996. (no. 49)

Authentic Movement: Essays by Mary Starks Whitehouse, Janet Adler and Joan Chodorow, Patrizia Pallaro (editor), Jessica Kingsley Publishers, London, 1999. (nos. 82, 130, 232, 309)

Autobiography of a Yogi, Paramahamsa Yogananda, Self-Realization Fellowship, Los Angeles, 1979. (no. 193)

Awakening the Buddha Within: Eight Steps to Enlightenment, Lama Surya Das, Broadway Books, New York, 1997 (no. 109)

Awakening the Spine, Vanda Scaravelli, Harper San Francisco, 1991. (nos. 164, 231, 308)

Ayurveda: Life, Health and Longevity, Robert E. Svoboda, Penguin Books, New Delhi, 1992. (nos. 147, 305)

Banaras, City of Light, Diana L. Eck, Princeton University Press, 1982. (nos. 218, 155)

Beyond God the Father: Toward a Philosophy of Women's Liberation, Mary Daly, Beacon Press, Boston, 1974. (no. 98)

Bhagavad Gita, Eknath Easwaran (translator), Nilgiri Press, Tomales, Calif., 1985. (nos. 114, 251)

Bhagavad Gita, Juan Moscaro (translator), Penguin Books, London, 1962. (nos. 54, 296, 270, 339, 344, 362)

Bhagavad Gita, Stephen Mitchell (translator), Three Rivers Press, New York, 2000. (nos. 15, 93, 284)

A Brief History of Everything, Ken Wilber, Shambhala, Boston and London, 1996. (no. 357)

By Means of Performance: Intracultural Studies of Theatre and Ritual, R. Schechner and W. Appel (editors), Cambridge University Press, Cambridge, 1990. (no. 174)

The Children of Barren Women, Pupul Jayakar, Penguin Books, India, 1994. (nos. 53, 241, 266)

Chinnamasta: The Aweful Buddhist and Hindu Tantric Goddess, Elisabeth Anne Benard, Motilal Barnarsidass, New Delhi, 1994. (no. 211)

Collected Shorter Plays (Footfalls), Samuel Beckett, Grove Press, New York, 1984. (no. 33)

The Collected Works of C. G. Jung, Princeton University Press, 1972. (no. 334)

Coming Home to Myself, Marion Woodman, Conari Press, Berkeley, Calif., 1998. (no. 31)

The Commentary on the Bowl of Saki of Hazrat Inayat Khan, Murshid Samuel Lewis, Sufi Islamia/Prophecy Publications, San Francisco, 1981. (no. 228)

The Complete Poems of Emily Dickinson, Emily Dickinson, Little, Brown, Boston, 1924. (no. 363)

The Conquest of Happiness, Bertrand Russell, George Allen and Unwin, London, 1975. (no. 44)

Consciousness Speaks, Conversations with Ramesh S. Balsekar, Wayne Liquorman (editor), Advaita Press, Redondo Beach, Calif., 1992. (nos. 80, 252, 310)

The Core of the Teachings, J. Krishnamurti, Krishnamurti Foundation Trust Ltd., 1980. (no. 86)

The Crescent Moon, Rabindranath Tagore, Macmillan, London, 1918. (nos. 223, 256)

Cutting Through Spiritual Materialism, Chogyam Trungpa, Shambhala, Boulder, Colo., 1973. (nos. 12, 157)

Drama Therapy with Families, Groups and Individuals: Waiting in the Wings, Sue Jennings, Jessica Kingsley Publishers, London, 1990. (no. 120)

Enjoyment of Laughter, Max Eastman, Johnson Reprint Corp, 1970. (no. 247)

The Essence of Yoga: Reflections on the Yoga Sutras of Patanjali, Bernard Bouanchaud, Rudra Press, Portland, Ore., 1997. (nos. 13, 261, 296, 317)

The Everyday Meditator, Osho, Charles E. Tuttle, Inc., Rutland, Vt., 1993. (no. 30)

Flowers from the Forest, Swami Nirmalananda, Vishwa Shanti Nikethana, B. R. Hills, India, 1991. (nos. 209, 265)

From Onions to Pearls, Satyam Nadeen, New Freedom Press, San Rafael, Calif., 1996. (no. 338)

Fundamentalism and the Middle Path, Richard Freeman, the Yoga Workshop, published on www.Yoga workshop.com, Boulder, Colo. No date given. (no. 213)

A Garland of Forest Flowers, Swami Nirmalananda, Vishwa Shanti Nikethana, B. R. Hills, India, 1993. (nos. 28, 72, 126, 352)

The Gift, Hafiz, Daniel Ladinsky (translator), Penguin/Compass, New York, 1999. (nos. 74, 201, 302)

God Bless the Child, Arthur Herzog, Jr., and Billie Holliday (composers), 1939. (no. 104)

Golden Nuggets, Bhagwan Shree Rajnesh (Osho), Rebel Publishing House, Cologne. No date given. (no. 165)

The Gospel of Sri Ramakrishna, Swami Nikhilananda (translator), Mylapore: Sri Ramakrishna Math, 1952. (nos. 88, 271, 283)

A Gradual Awakening, Stephen Levine, Anchor Books, New York, 1979. (nos. 78, 273)

Grist for the Mill, Ram Dass, Celestial Arts, Berkeley, 1976. (nos. 43, 170)

The Hatha Yoga Pradipika, Pancham Singh, Sri Satguru Publications, New Delhi, 1915. (nos. 222, 329, 355)

The Hatha Yoga Pradipika, Yoga Swami Svatmarama, Elsy Becherer (translator), Aquarian/Thorsons, 1972. (nos. 7, 69, 100, 342)

Healing Mantras, Thomas Ashley-Farrand, Ballantine Wellspring, New York, 1999. (no. 6: mantra translation only, 121)

Health, Healing and Beyond: Yoga and the Living Tradition of Krishnamacharya, T. K. V. Desikachar and R. H. Cravens, Aperture, New York, 1998. (nos. 156, 203)

Hidden Journey: A Spirtual Awakening, Andrew Harvey, Arkana/Penguin, New York, 1992. (no. 205)

Hinduism, Louis Renou (editor), George Braziller, New York, 1962. (nos. 277, 347)

Hindu Scriptures, Dominic Goodall (translator), University of California Press, Berkeley, 1996. (no. 184)

A Hole Is to Dig, Ruth Krauss, HarperTrophy, New York, reprint edition 1989. (no. 255)

How to Know God: The Yoga Aphorisms of Patanjali, Swami Prabhavananda and Christopher Isherwood, New American Library, New York, 1953. (nos. 169, 175, 235, 335)

How We Live Our Yoga, Valerie Jeremijenko (editor), Beacon Press, Boston, 2001. (no. 238)

Hymns to the Goddess, Sir John Woodroffe, Ganesh and Co, Madras, India, 1913. (nos. 17, 131, 162)

I Am That: Talks with Sri Nisargadatta Maharaj, Sudhaker S. Dikshit (editor), Aperture, New York, 1997. (nos. 5, 142)

Inner Revolution, Robert Thurman, Riverhead Books, New York, 1998. (nos. 141, 303)

In the Dark of the Heart, Songs of Meera, Shama Futehally (translator), HarperCollins, New York, 1994. (no. 111)

Invocation to Patanjali, B. K. S. Iyengar (translator). Date and publisher unknown. (no. 1)

Isavasya Upanishad, Swami Chinmayananda (translator), Central Chinmaya Mission Trust, Mumbai, India, 1997. (no. 62)

Jivamukti Yoga, Practices for Liberating Body and Soul, Sharon Gannon and David Life, Ballantine Books, New York, 2002. (nos. 37, 287)

Ka, Roberto Calasso, Tim Parks (translator), Vintage Books, New York, 1998. (nos. 56, 132)

Kamakala Chidvalli in Kali: The Feminine Force, Ajit Mookerjee, Destiny Books, Rochester, Vt., 1988. (no. 354)

The Kamasutra for Women, Vinod Verma, Kodansha America, New York, 1997. (no. 336)

Kundalini, Path to Higher Consciousness, Gopi Krishna, Orient Paperbacks, New Delhi, 1992. (no. 41)

Life Ahead, J. Krishnamurti, HarperCollins, New York, February 1975. (no. 127)

The Little Book of Questions, U. G. Krishnamurti, Penguin Books, India, 2000. (nos. 69, 138, 297)

The Little Prince, Antoine de Saint-Exupéry, Harcourt Paperbacks, New York (1943 original), reprint edition 2000. (no. 194)

Living at the Source: Yoga Teachings of Vivekananda, Ann Myren and Dorothy Madison Shambhala (editors), Boston, 1993. (nos. 38, 107, 206, 327)

Living Within, The Yoga Approach to Psychological Health and Growth, Sri Aurobindo Ashram Trust, Pondicherry, India, 1987. (nos. 18, 66, 101, 353)

Maharshi's Gospel: The Teachings of Sri Ramana Maharshi, Venkataraman, Tiruvannamalai, India, 1969. (nos. 153, 294, 337)

Martin Luther King, Arnold Michaelis (interviewer), University of Georgia and the Martin Luther King, Jr., Center for Nonviolent Social Change, Inc., 1967. (nos. 148, 285)

Meditations and Mantras, Swami Vishnu Devananda, Om Oltus Publishing, New York, 1978. (no. 246 with my own translation)

Memories, Dreams, Reflections, C. G. Jung, Routledge & Keegan, London, 1963. (nos. 89, 262)

The Mysticism of Sound and Music, Hazrat Inayat Khan, Shambhala, Boston, 1996. (nos. 52, 159)

My Three Reasons for Hope, Jane Goodall, the Jane Goodall Institute, Silver Spring, Md., 2001. (no. 75)

Neem Karoli Baba Web Site: www.neemkaroli.com, 1999–2003. (no. 318, 341)

"No Independent Existence, an Interview with the Dalai Lama," Amy Edelstein in *What Is Enlightenment?* Issue 17, fall/winter 1999. (no. 22)

Ocean of Sound (Ocean of Silence), Sri Karunamayee talks to Marcus Boon in *Ascent* magazine, Timeless Books, issue 14, summer, Montreal, 2002. (nos. 71, 216)

One Day My Soul Just Opened Up, Iyanla Vanzant, Simon & Schuster, New York, 1998. (no. 64)

One Hundred Poems of Kabir, Rabindranath Tagore and Evelyn Underhill (translators), Macmillan India, 1915. (nos. 144, 263, 280, 314)

On Love and Loneliness, J. Krishnamurti, Harper San Francisco, 1993. (no. 288)

On Love, Sri Aurobindo and the Mother, Pavitra (editor), Sri Aurobindo Ashram Trust, Pondicherry, India, 1966. (no. 237)

Our Inner Conflicts: A Constructive Theory of Neurosis, Karen Horney, W. W. Norton, New York, reissue edition 1993. (no. 145)

Patanjali's Yoga Sutras, An Introduction, T. K. V. Desikacher, Affiliated East-West Press PVT, Ltd., Madras, India, 1987. (no. 97)

The Path of Practice: Healing with Food, Breath and Sound, Bri Maya Tiwari, Ballantine, New York, 2000. (nos. 122, 244, 312)

Poems (unpublished), Jonathan Lewis, 2002. Used by permission of author. (nos. 150, 326)

The Prophet, Kahlil Gibran, Knopf, New York, 1923. (nos. 177, 293)

Rappaport, Julie. (nos. 3, 6, 8, 11, 14, 16, 19, 22, 26, 29, 32, 35, 39, 42, 46, 51, 57, 58, 67, 73, 76, 83, 85, 87, 91, 96, 99, 102, 106, 112, 116, 123, 125, 128, 133, 136, 140, 143, 149, 151, 158, 161, 168, 171, 176, 179, 182, 183, 188, 192, 195, 199, 204, 207, 210, 215, 220, 225, 226, 227, 233, 236, 239, 243, 245, 248, 250, 254, 255, 258, 260, 264, 268, 269, 274, 276, 282, 286, 290, 295, 298, 301, 313, 319, 321, 323, 325, 328, 330, 333, 340, 348, 350, 354, 358, 364)

Reflections, Walter Benjamin, Schocken Books, New York, 1986. (no. 154)

Re-Visioning Psychology, James Hillman, Harper Perennial, New York, 1992. (nos. 9, 115)

The River Below, François Cheng, Welcome Rain, New York, 2000. (no. 113)

"The Room Before Paradise," Swami Rudrananda, in *Rudra,* March 1983, Nityananda Institute, Portland, Ore. (no. 240)

Science Order, and Creativity: A Dramatic New Look at the Creative Roots of Science and Life, David Bohm, Bantam, New York, reissue edition 1987. (no. 55)

Sensing, Feeling and Action, Bonnie Bainbridge-Cohen, Contact Editions, Northampton, Mass., 1993. (no. 20)

Silence, John Cage, Wesleyan University Press, Middletown, Conn., 1961. (nos. 50, 224)

Siva Samhita, Rai Bahadur Srisa Chandra Vasu (translator), Allhabad, India, 1914. (nos. 81, 124, 178, 322)

The Soul Would Have No Rainbow If the Eyes Had No Tears, Guy A. Zona, Touchstone, New York, 1994 (no. 306)

A Source Book in Indian Philosophy, Sarvepalli Radhakrishnan and Charles A. Moore (editors), Princeton University Press, 1957. (nos. 198, 365)

Source Book of Ancient Indian Psychology, B. Kuppuswamy (editor), Konark Publishers, Delhi, 1993. (nos. 160, 356)

Sri Aurobindo: A Greater Psychology, A. S. Dalal (editor), Tarcher/Putnam, New York, 2001. (nos. 24, 105)

Sri Krishnamacharya: The Purnacarya, Krishnamacharya Yoga Mandiram, Madras, India, 1997. (no. 25)

Swami Dayananda Saraswati Lectures, held at Arsha Vidya Gurukulam, Saylorsburg, Pa., 2003. (nos. 189, 208, 242)

Sweet on My Lips: The Love Poems of Mirabai, Louise Landes Levi, Cool Grove Press, New York, 1997. (no. 103)

Taittiriya Upanishad, Swami Chinmayananda, Central Chinmayananda Mission Trust, Bombay, 1992. (nos. 3, 279)

A Tale of Two Gardens, Octavio Paz, Viking/Penguin, India, 1997. (nos. 40, 180)

The Tantric Way, Ajit Mookerjee and Madhu Khanna, Thames and Hudson, London, 1997. (no. 197)

The Tao of Leadership, Lao Tzu's Tao Te Ching Adapted for a New Age, John Heider, Humanics Publishing Group, Lake Worth, Fla., 1986. (no. 36)

There Is No Natural Religion, William Blake (c. 1788 original), The William Blake Archive, Morris Eaves, Robert N. Essick, and Joseph Viscomi (editors), the Institute for Advanced Technology in the Humanities, www.blake archive.org, 1996–2002. (nos. 117, 349)

The Thirteen Principal Upanishads, R. E. Hume (translator), Oxford University Press, London, 1921. (nos. 44, 278)

Thoughts and Aphorisms, Sri Aurobindo Trust, Pondicherry, India, 1958. (nos. 253, 304)

The Tibetan Book of Living and Dying, Sogyal Rinpoche, Harper San Francisco, 1992. (nos. 219, 259, 343)

The Tree of Knowledge, Humberto Maturana, Francisco Varela, Shambala, Boston and London, 1992. (no. 146)

The Tree of Yoga, B. K. S. Iyengar, Shambhala, Boston, 1989. (nos. 23, 167)

The Upanishads, Eknath Easwaran (translator), Nilgiri Press, Tomales, Calif., 1987. (nos. 47, 77, 317)

The Upanishads, Swami Paramananda, Project Gutenberg Archive, 2002, Oxford, Miss. (nos. 160, 170, 331)

The Upanishads, volumes 1 and 2, F. Max Muller (translator), Oxford University Press, 1884. (nos. 70, 360, 267)

Vasishta's Yoga, Swami Venkatesananda (translator), State University of New York Press, Albany, 1993. (nos. 2, 234, 324, 346, 359)

Viveka Chudamani, Adi Sankara, Bharata Iyer (compiler), Bombay, 1982. (no. 129)

Wake Up and Roar, Satang with H. W. L. Poonja, vol. 1, Eli Jaxon-Bear (editor), Pacific Center Press, Maui, 1992. (nos. 34, 137)

"When You Go Beyond the Ego, You Become an Offering to the World," interview with Mata Amritanandamayi by Amy Edelstein in *What Is Enlightenment?* Issue 17, fall/winter 1999. (no. 214)

Wherever You Go, There You Are: Mindfulness Meditation in Everyday Life, Jon Kabat-Zinn, Hyperion, New York, 1995. (no. 140)

William James Site: www. emory.deu/education/mfp/james.html (no. 345)

The Wisdom of Insecurity, Alan W. Watts, Vintage, New York, 1951. (nos. 90, 202)

The Words of Gandhi, Richard Attenborough, Newmarket Press, New York, 1982. (no. 48)

A Year in Thoreau's Journal, 1851, Henry David Thoreau, Penguin Classics, New York, 1993. (no. 65)

Yoga: Discipline of Freedom, The Yoga Sutra Attributed to Patanjali, Barbara Stoler Miller, University of California Press, Berkeley, 1995. (nos. 152, 191)

Yoga: The Spirit and Practice of Moving into Stillness, Erich Schiffmann, Pocket Books, New York, 1996. (nos. 289, 361)

The Yoga and Its Objects, Sri Aurobindo Ashram, Pondicherry 1921. (no. 4)

Yoga and the Hindu Tradition (Siva Samhita), Jean Varenne (translator), University of Chicago Press, 1976. (no. 10)

"Yoga as Transformation," Joel Kramer, *Yoga Journal*, Berkeley, Calif., May/June 1980. (nos. 59, 249)

Yoga for Body, Breath and Mind, A. G. Mohan, Rudra Press Cambridge, Mass., 1993. (no. 300)

Yoga Immortality and Freedom, Mircea Eliade, Princeton University Press, 1969. (no. 173)

Yoganjalisaram, Krishnamacharya Granthamala, Krishnamacharya Yoga Mandiram, Madras, 1995. (no. 108)

Yoga of Heart: The Healing Power of Intimate Connection, Mark Whitwell, Lantern Books, New York, 2004. (nos. 118, 163, 272)

A Yoga of Indian Classical Dance: The Yogini's Mirror, Roxanne Kamayani Gupta, Inner Traditions, Rochester, Vt., 2000. (nos. 166, 327)

The Yoga of Spiritual Devotion: A Modern Translation of the Bhakti Narada Sutras, Prem Prakash, Inner Traditions, Rochester, Vt., 1998. (nos. 28, 92, 187)

The Yoga of T. Krishnamacharya, T. K. V. Desikachar, KYM Publishers, Madras, India, 1989. (no. 61)

The Yoga Sutras of Patanjali, Sri Swami Satchidananda, Integral Yoga Publications, Yogaville, Va., 1999. (no. 181)

ACKNOWLEDGMENTS

I would like to thank the following people for helping me to shape this book: Pranams go out to my agent, Stephany Evans, for her assistance throughout the hunting, gathering, and writing phases; my editor at Tarcher/Penguin, Sara Carder, for her enthusiasm for both this project and yoga; Jonathan Lewis for permission to use his poems and valuable feedback; Will Paice, Laura Y. Rappaport, Joan Allekotte and family, Terese Gjernes, and Ashley Sharpe for text support; Patty Phelps for photo support, the yoga students of Berkeley, San Francisco, and Yoga Bliss for your helpful reflections and dedication; Sri Karunamayee for spiritual guidance, music, and words; Anja Borgstrom and Amber Lotus Publishers for inviting me into the yoga-writing-art synthesis; to all my yoga gurus past, present, and future for the gift of your teachings; and to my loving circle of friends and family who have supported me throughout this process: *Namaste.*

ABOUT THE AUTHOR

A student of yoga since 1986, Julie Rappaport is a yoga teacher and writer based in the San Francisco Bay Area. She is the founder and director of Yoga Bliss and offers international yoga workshops and retreats.

Julie also holds advanced clinical degrees in psychology and drama therapy and maintains a private practice in yoga therapy and mind-body–centered psychotherapy.

For information about her programs, she can be reached through her Web site: www.yogabliss.com.